A Food is Medicine RD® Book

in the PINK

A Breast Cancer Survivor's Guide to a Healthier Life

Laurie Hatch, RD
Breast Cancer Survivor and
Registered Cancer Dietitian

Cover designs and book illustrations by Betty Lok, Betty Wonderful, LLC, www.bettywonderful.com

Edited by Alexandra O'Connell, Your Resident Wordsmith LLC

Cover and interior design by Victoria Wolf, wolfdesignandmarketing.com

ISBN 979-8-9873375-2-3 (eBook)
ISBN 979-8-9873375-0-9 (Paperback)

Printed in U. S. A.

Published by Food Is Medicine RD Books, LLC
Brighton, Colorado

2024

www.foodismedicinerd.com

I can do all things through Christ who strengthens me.
—Philippians 4:13

CONTENTS

PREFACE

ONE IN EIGHT AMERICAN WOMEN will receive a breast cancer diagnosis during her lifetime. The median age at diagnosis is sixty-two. Two-thirds of the diagnoses will be estrogen-positive breast cancer. Over 90 percent will survive five years and many beyond.[1] Top-notch cancer care has resulted in cure rates unheard of for other cancers. Many studies demonstrate that better eating habits, moderate weight loss, and more physical activity prevent the risk of recurrence, adding quality to the years of a survivor's life. This is great news. But what I have witnessed repeatedly is that upon completion of treatment, survivors experience a lack of education and support to help them establish healthier habits. Improved eating habits and more physical movement are only minimally addressed. Resources to foster better lifestyle activities need a personalized flair for the wide variety of survivors' nutritional needs and physical abilities.

After my diagnosis of breast cancer in 2014 at the age of fifty-two, and following a decade working in cancer care as a registered dietitian, I became a member of the pink-crazed Breast Cancer Club. As a result of my work, I was familiar with the exquisitely personal experience that women have with their diagnosis and treatment. What I did not appreciate until my own diagnosis was the struggle to reclaim health following treatment. Having professionally delved into how eating and exercise can impact the health of breast cancer survivors, I knew the price to pay if I did not work toward managing my lifestyle habits with greater attention. I wanted to change my imperfect habits *right now.* And I tried, more than once, during my treatment and immediately at the end, to do just that. But I was not ready. I was woefully slapdash in my attempts to eat better or resume physical activity. I was disgusted with my lapsed health habits. How could I join the Breast Cancer Club when a gray fog hung over me in my sadness?

What I lacked was personal grace and the right brand of motivation. I was accustomed to pushing my way through daily habits with a heavy hand, getting instant results. What I needed was a softer touch, like that of a feather, to change my habits a little at a time in step with my emotions. I began to see the same need in other breast cancer survivors. Each of us shines with our own shade of pink. Some glow fuchsia reflecting passionate triumph over the disease. Others show a softer tone of ballet slipper or bubblegum pink, suggesting a more bashful style. My early shade of pink was more coral than pink, reflecting my smoldering scorn toward my plight. Regardless of the shade of pink on display, we need delicacy, a lighter touch that will urge us onward to a healthier life. After treatment, we need more grace and less haste.

What survivors receive from their cancer care team is heartfelt and proven advice about nutrition and physical activity. Absent is concrete guidance, like what to do, how to begin safely, and how to stay motivated. Food and nutrition questions arise but are addressed with a boilerplate handout or, worse, answered by misinformation in the press or among acquaintances. Notably, this book cannot address individual lifestyle needs or treat disease, but it does answer frequently asked questions, tell stories about other survivors, provide science-based direction about the importance of lifestyle changes, give tips on how to trade unfavorable habits for better ones, and present evidence-based nutrition information benefiting breast cancer survivors. It is designed as a source of information and education for the early-stage (0–3) survivor with cancer that has not spread to distant organs or tissues. It guides a survivor to begin a better eating style or safely increase physical activity.

I attest to the fact that breast cancer survivors do not receive the kind of support they need to lead them toward a healthier life. I spent sixteen years working in cancer care, but the hours devoted to breast cancer survivors were minor compared to the amount of time spent addressing the nutritional needs of patients with cancers of the lung, head and neck, colon, and stomach. Patients with these diagnoses lose weight drastically and cannot eat, which threatens their ability to continue to receive treatments that save their lives. These patients required most of my efforts. I was unable to provide the time, attention, and ability to be present when these women needed me most.

In the last five years of my work in cancer care, I found a way to gather breast cancer survivors into a program and seize upon their desire to work their way toward greater health. Educational guidance, tailored to their needs, included weight loss, plant-based diets, physical activity, and bone health—the same education that is tucked into the chapters of this book and in the companion journal. Over fifty women participated in my lifestyle group, and each of them brought their own stories. Some were younger than fifty; others were well into their seventies. One was both grandma and mom to several children while working full time with scant financial resources. Most of them were fifty-five and over. Several had triple-negative breast cancer; one had experienced two recurrences. A handful had diabetes, while one or two had heart disease after treatment. Our group was focused on weight loss, and the average loss was fifteen pounds. Two lost more than forty pounds in a year. I am proud of what they accomplished. I would not have missed doing this for the world, and some of their stories are in this book. Their names have been changed to protect their privacy.

With the right information and guidance, good health is restored. My survivors showed me that this works. Yet my research for this book showed that despite emerging evidence and professional guidance for improved eating patterns, better food choices, and consistent exercise, programs aimed at survivors are not yet a standard of care.

The situation is changing slowly as reimbursement for cancer exercise programming and dedicated nutritional services for survivors improves, but this is going to take time. Meanwhile, I decided to write this book. The research for this book and the companion journal is based on my personal experience and my years of working with survivors as a dietitian. I know what scares you about food, and I know where to look for the answers to take down the fear. I know where you hurt when you try to move more and sit less, so I look for ways to safely get you started. I know that you are bitter and confused, and so I lead you gently toward your own motivation within your capabilities and desires. Because of my personal and professional insights, I chose to get the word out about how small but impactful changes can enhance the lives of many survivors.

There is more to moving a survivor forward than educating them about nutrition concepts or presenting generic advice. Each survivor and her story is unique. Some women feel a triumph of having endured treatment, while others experience defeat and sadness. I became aware of fellow survivors who appeared to pause when the hard feelings bubbled up, as if to say, *Wait a minute, there is something else going on here.* I observed how some of them, regardless of their feelings of triumph or defeat, became grateful for the miracle of medicine, the tender touch of family and friends, and a smiling radiation tech. I want more breast cancer survivors to arrive at a place where they recognize that their experience with breast cancer does not have to keep them from restoring their health. But, this part of the cancer experience cannot be done alone. You need guidance, and you want to do more than survive; you want to thrive.

Enduring cancer treatment is no simple task, but neither is revamping diet or exercise habits. Light and subtle changes form healthier habits one small detail at a time, simple strokes of brilliance that change the mind and body until you are "in the pink," or at the pinnacle of health.

Finally, I believe in bringing truth to nutrition and genuine guidance to breast cancer survivors all over. This book is written to tell the breast cancer survivor that grand lifestyle changes are not needed. The companion journal is designed to allow you to reflect on current habits at your own pace. And this is what cancer food and nutrition experts know: small changes to food choices and physical activity have been proven by numerous studies to give durable health benefits. Survivors need a toolbox filled with useful, expert guidance and answers to questions. When you are ready to get started, fair survivor, keep this in mind: begin with an attitude of gratitude.

Laurie Hatch

INTRODUCTION

SURVIVORS OF BREAST CANCER carry considerable emotional trauma into and beyond treatment. Shock becomes anger, and sadness enhances depression as the emotional toll evolves over the course of diagnosis. Surprisingly, starting treatment brings calm; once you know you have cancer, you want to start the process of destroying it. With treatment underway, you grow calmer, as cancer is being handled by experts. A calendar filled with appointments brings relief, with opportunities to visit the doctors and nurses who provide encouragement and hope. Through chemo and radiation, you count the days until you are done. You fantasize about the end of treatment, certain that all will return to normal. But as treatment completion draws near, an inexplicable anxiety emerges. You wonder, *How will I get my life back?*

Helping you do so—filling in the gaps between completing treatment and restoring your health and hope—are the goals of this book. Professionally, I have been aware of the need to address the desires of breast cancer survivors since 2004, when I began my role as a cancer dietitian. Out of the gate, I botched my first presentation with breast cancer survivors who were seeking answers to nutrition questions. All I could come up with was a well-phrased recommendation to eat more high-antioxidant blueberries and lose a little weight. The emotional upheaval of this cancer escaped me, as did the need to dig a little deeper and understand what I could offer beyond a cup of blueberries. Years later, and with hundreds of consultations with breast cancer survivors under my belt, I knew there had to be a better way.

In 2010, I was asked to speak at a cancer dietitian's conference in Connecticut about the possibility of insurance billing and coding for cancer survivorship visits. My dietitian colleagues and I were giddy about the prospect of getting survivorship visits with a dietitian, a social worker, and a doctor or nurse reimbursed by insurance. Research that I used at the time for my presentation supported the idea that insurance reimbursement for these visits was on the horizon with the Affordable Care Act (ACA). Prior to the implementation of the ACA in 2013, there was a glimmer of hope that survivorship visits would be covered under this legislation, like other chronic diseases. To date, this has not happened. A National Cancer Resource Center was created in 2013, and while this group has made progress, much of it has been in gathering evidence on whether survivorship visits are cost-effective, figuring out the details of which medical professionals will be responsible and what type of services will be covered.[2] For now, survivorship visits are not fully covered by insurance, and many services will require co-pays or coinsurance. The cost of a healthy survivorship is an ongoing expense for several years.[3]

It has been more than thirteen years since my presentation to other cancer dietitians, and while more evidence in support of nutritional and physical activity guidance emerges, there is still no clear-cut way to get insurance coverage for survivorship care, specifically for nutrition visits. Nonetheless, a consultation with a cancer dietitian is available upon request in many cancer centers across the US; all you need to do is ask your doctor. To address survivors' needs, many cancer dietitians and nurse navigators valiantly attempt to meet the demand with classes, programs, presentations, and basic leaflets. Too often, though, these attempts fall short of the fervent requests for the supportive guidance needed to truly help. Cancer dietitians carry a heavy patient load and struggle to address these requests with the attention every patient wants and needs. The painful truth is that survivorship guidance is still in the hands and pocketbooks of survivors. Due to the financial toxicity associated with treatment co-pays, imaging bills, missed work, and other expenses, paying for dietitian visits, gym memberships, diet programs, or personal trainers is often out of reach.

Several years ago, a new requirement to provide survivors with a Survivorship Care Plan, a document organizing information about follow-up care, the types of tests needed in years to come, and the potential long-term late effects of cancer treatments, became mandatory. Suggestions for healthy living, such as getting more physically active or improving one's eating pattern, are included in the care plan document.[4] Some cancer centers make strong efforts to help survivors with generic information and referrals to community-based social workers and dietitians, but too often, survivors navigate their return to a healthier life alone. Some larger university-based cancer centers offer survivorship visits with a team comprised of social workers, dietitians, and a doctor or nurse, during which a personal plan for emotional, social, nutritional, and medical health needs is addressed.

My diagnosis in 2014 changed my approach; it was humbling to sit among the survivors I helped while waiting in the queue for my own treatments. Moments perched on the benches, dressed in my treatment gown, allowed time to rethink what I really knew about cancer survivorship and, more importantly, what I was going to do about it. Underneath it all, a plan was growing.

In the Pink began as notes scribbled on scrap paper, notes about what breast cancer survivors want and need to know about restoring their health. Thousands of my pink sisters had proven to me that simply sharing a meal plan, a diet, an instruction sheet on antioxidants, and a talk about soy and low-fat foods was inadequate. The reality of my breast cancer diagnosis enlightened me; there is more to helping a survivor than a few hastily scrawled recommendations. You need gentleness, a softer touch, and small nutritional corrections with no scolding. This book acknowledges that while your toughness is a given, my compassion is essential.

Because I am aware of the strong emotional price breast cancer exacts on you and me, I recognize the value of the practice of gratitude as the starting place. And so, the first chapter, "An Attitude of Gratitude," explores how gratitude helps you make sense of how cancer has changed you, how to find peace in the present, and finally, how to create a vision for a healthier future. Far too many survivors apologize for old habits that have not served them well, habits like too much junk food, sitting for hours each day without a walk, or skipping breakfast, but I firmly believe it is never too late to trade these old ways for better ones. Chapter 2, "Trade Old Habits for Better Ones," shows there is no quick fix for adopting new habits, but with the perseverance you acquired while getting through treatment, you have the right stuff to do so.

Take the time to reflect on the first two chapters, as they set the stage for those that follow. "Food as Medicine" provides a nutritional foundation with clear details about how the food you eat acts as medicine as nutrients restore and maintain health. That chapter leads to "Puzzle Pieces," which explores the connections between breast cancer, heart disease, and diabetes. Using nutritional puzzle pieces, you learn how to arrange nutrients through healthy eating patterns to manage or prevent these diseases.

Physical activity, or the dreaded word "exercise," is not a nutritional component, but it is strong medicine, too. Chapter 5, "Glisten," presents a new way to approach physical activity, beginning with short bouts and building up to doable amounts that accomplish much, especially when combined with a healthier way of eating. As a fan of William Shakespeare and his clever twist of words, I could not resist using "In the Pink" as both a chapter title and the name of the book. To be at the pinnacle of health is to be "in the pink." Years of receiving requests from survivors on how to get their lives back suggests to me that people like you wish to, once again, be in tip-top shape. Chapter 6, the book's namesake chapter, goes deeper into evidence-based studies supporting specific nutrients that enhance the health of breast cancer survivors while stressing the importance of making every bit of food count. Finally, chapter 7, "A Brighter Shade of Pink," includes my creation, the In the Pink Plate Plan, an eating plan adapted from the Dietary Guidelines for Americans and further devised with seven groups of foods given priority for breast cancer survivors. In fact, as I reflect on the many survivor visits conducted throughout my career, I wish I could have more completely emphasized the significance these seven food groups have on survivor health.

Finally, the accompanying *In the Pink: Companion Journal* serves as your private place to reflect on your readiness to make lifestyle changes, practice self-affirming phrases, take an honest look at eating habits, create goals for improved food choices, and more. Beautifully and playfully designed, the pages are inviting and thought-provoking.

My cancer diagnosis knocked me to my knees so much that, perhaps like you, I reached the bottom, not knowing what my life would be like from that point on. What emerged was a far-reaching decision to move 2,500 miles across the country from New England and back to my hometown in Colorado. After getting settled, I returned to work in a cancer center near my home in 2016. I walked through those doors with the precious knowledge of the physical and emotional toll of this disease. For five years, I performed as both a dietitian and a cancer survivor; the lessons could not have been more heartrending. For the first time, I felt what you felt. I was changed and better for it.

In 2021, I left this position and, seven months later, I created the outline for *In the Pink*. This book, and the accompanying journal, is the culmination of my unique viewpoint in these two roles. It is my sincere attempt to give you a framework that fills the gaps between what you want to know, the guidance you desire, and the level of help you receive.

More than ever before, I am aware of the growing body of evidence over the last twenty years that suggests diet, regular physical activity, and a normal body weight improve breast cancer outcomes, which means healthier, longer lives for you and me.[5] I also know that nutritional consultations, gym memberships, deliveries of packaged weight loss foods, and other promises for healthier lives that are peddled everywhere can be out of reach. My two books were created with this in mind because I understand that while the initial purchase is considerable, the cost is well below other services available to you.

Most breast cancer survivors have estrogen-positive cancer, but as you will see, concepts presented in this book lead you to a healthier life, regardless of whether your cancer is estrogen-positive or negative. I hope you understand you are not your unhealthy habits, and trading undesired habits for better ones is possible, even if you have had an unhealthy habit for a long time. My desire is that you recognize the resiliency that has been with you all along. For those of you who have devoted your lives to the care of others, I desire that you discover that your self-care is more than worth the trouble.

Finishing the book before you begin to change your habits is not necessary. Begin where you are today. Use a light touch, like a feather, to form a healthier future by beginning with a daily gratitude offering to set a positive tone in mood and action. Or choose to eat five servings of vegetables and fruits daily, as this food group offers more disease-fighting components than the other groups. Try getting up out of the chair three times a day to dance or march in five-minute bouts to strengthen your heart, calm your mind, and boost your metabolism. The guidance in the book should feel like an invitation to paint your healthier future on a canvas with a feather, not bang it back together with a hammer.

CHAPTER 1

An Attitude of Gratitude

"Gratitude makes sense of our past, brings peace
for today, and creates a vision for tomorrow."

—MELODY BEATTIE

WITH THE REASSURANCE of a clean mammogram and a doctor's blessing, you survive, but at a price. On the outside, you look fine to family, friends, and co-workers. They nod at you reassuringly when they hear that treatment is completed. But on the inside, corners of you are slow to heal. A breast cancer diagnosis upends how you feel, how you see yourself, and what thoughts fill your head. Your body will never be quite the same. Your mind is troubled with relapse worries, and your joy is stolen. You feel stuck, even trapped, by what you now carry. How do you set this burden down and begin again?

Years ago, many cancer survivors felt alone in the emotional struggles with their disease, but today, research offers evidence-based guidance about the power of gratefulness and affirming self-talk that lifts the moods and, with that, activities of survivors. Today, it is well-accepted that you can do more than survive; you can thrive, but you need some direction. Based on evidence, experts know that minor shifts in your thoughts, emotions, and feelings can add up to bringing you peace and hope for the future. In this chapter, you will explore how to:

- Begin with gratitude.
- Think more positively.
- Recognize your resilient spirit.
- Talk to yourself with love and admiration.

This is where you start to rid your life of the untidy heap left over from diagnosis and treatment. Within this chapter, I introduce you to your own resiliency and invite you to explore and practice gratitude. You will gain an understanding of your why, your purpose, and how this motivates you, bestowing on you the confidence you need to get down to building new habits for a healthier life. Through gratitude and a resilient spirit, you move toward greater healing.

Gratitude Moves You toward Healing

Gratitude is broadly defined as the appreciation of what is valuable and meaningful to oneself. It also represents a general state of thankfulness. Some say gratitude is a moral virtue; others see it as an attitude or a habit. Still others say it is an emotion or a personality trait. Practicing gratitude as you received treatment entailed a dependency on your treatment team, family members, friends, or neighbors. An appreciation for those who helped you through treatment plants seeds for improving your health while also fostering in you a desire for helping others. Simply stated, gratitude fosters the desire to pay it forward. Gratitude nourishes these seeds of hope, setting up new possibilities. Generally, the act of gratitude involves a dependence on the kindness and generosity of others.[6]

Still, some people are uncomfortable with the obligatory aspect of gratitude. Before my cancer, I doubted the wisdom of gratitude. I did not believe that an attitude of gratitude gave someone tools to change. And gratefulness after cancer seemed a ridiculous proposal. Regardless of how you define or perceive it, though, studies show gratitude helps you thrive.

In 2010, researchers Emmons and McCullough looked at the impact that a conscious focus on blessings, or gratefulness, has on happiness and well-being.[7] To test this, they created three groups of participants who would all journal about an assigned condition. The first group focused their writing on gratitude during a hassle or negative life event. The second group journaled only about a hassle. The third group wrote down an account of each day's events. Results of the study showed that the gratitude group was more optimistic about the future, had fewer symptoms of physical illness, and spent significantly more time exercising than the other two groups.

My cancer diagnosis altered my frame of mind. Gratitude was the place I had to begin so that I could cast off physical and mental obstacles. Whatever limitations I was holding on to, I did not wish to keep them. I began to view my cancer through a lens of possibility, and not just for me. I was thinking about you. *How do I shift the perspective of fellow survivors and use it to guide them toward a healthier life?* Instead of inquiring about nutrition goals, I could begin by asking: "What brings you joy?"

You may cock your head to the side when I ask about what brings you joy. A common response is: "Excuse me? Joy for what? Cancer is awful! My joy has been stolen." It is crazy to think about joy, never mind gratitude, after cancer. But we all yearn for good health, a loving family, and hope for the future. Though simple and possibly overstated these days, a regular practice of gratitude allows us to make sense of what happened as we went through cancer treatment. It brings peace to us as we give thanks for the small stuff that rises to greet us. Gratitude gives us the horizon that holds the dream of our future. Slowly, you shed the raw, negative emotions of cancer therapy. Through gratitude and a resilient spirit, you move toward greater healing.

On the heels of gratitude come the joy and laughter you missed. It may surprise you at first, but the reappearance of joy means you are letting in positivity and hope. A decision has been made to behave in a positive manner to events around you, serving as a beacon of understanding that you find yourself worth it. Soon you are asking yourself how, by changing the frame around your cancer, you can recognize the triumph you displayed while getting through treatment.

Gratitude assists in removing the negative and replacing it with positive thoughts, feelings, and actions. This seems strange at first, perhaps even phony, and while not impossible, it does require important work in the mind and heart. Practicing gratitude drowns out the voice inside that spouts off negativity, telling you that you are not enough, you will fail, or that no one cares. Practicing gratitude tells you there are better things around the next corner.

Accordingly, I encourage you to open each day with a habit of practicing gratitude. I offer the following ways to begin fitting gratitude and positivity into your days:

- Express gratitude daily for the smallest of blessings.
- Visualize yourself taking excellent care of your mind and body.
- Focus on the freedom to choose what you desire for your health.
- Accept and expect that positive changes are just around the corner.
- Journal about things for which you are grateful. Send a note of thanks to someone.

To move toward more positive thinking is to lay the groundwork for getting your life back. I am not dismissing the challenges and struggles of breast cancer. But embracing gratitude must come before making a list of any new health habits you are considering. Sadness stalls our efforts to take better care of ourselves. Anger leads to frustration. Fear causes you to freeze in your tracks; you are afraid of any slight misstep. Confusion dwells in the mix of emotions, making you feel buried by the negative thoughts playing like a song stuck in your head. Gratitude quells the fear, anger, sadness, and confusion that cancer brings. Gratitude brings peace and a mindful presence, and it frames the vision for your future. It allows you to sit quietly to meditate on what you have endured, offer thanks to the people who helped you, and appreciate the small stuff.

Specifically, these phrases are a starting point to enhance feelings of gratitude:

- "I am grateful for another chance to live my life."
- "I am so grateful for the people I have in my life."
- "I am grateful for who I am and what I have."
- "Even though it is painful, I am grateful for the stones of hardship."
- "I am grateful to be growing stronger because of life's challenges."

The tussle with cancer is real, and cuddling with gratitude is vital to how you live going forward. I am in this club with you. I am uniquely positioned to cajole you with this. I am no longer a cancer dietitian, looking in from the outside, telling people what they should do to eat better without understanding what they have experienced. Not only have I witnessed the trauma of breast cancer in my work, but I have also experienced it, and I know what you have faced. I know what you can do, and I identify with the work to be done to claim a healthy future.

When I returned to working as a cancer dietitian after my treatment, and then as I wrote this book, I realized that our healthier lives are not just about eating better, exercising more, and losing weight. Further, I recognized that none of us can launch into a new eating plan, exercise regimen, or weight-loss program until the heavy emotional toll is honestly addressed. We must start at the beginning by acknowledging our hurts, practicing gratitude for our lives, and healing the raw corners of our minds and hearts. Only then can we get on our way to building the habits that will nudge us toward greater health.

My Cancer Story Began with Tears

Yours did, too. As a cancer dietitian, I thought my own diagnosis might imply that I was not particularly good at what I do. The day I received my diagnosis, I curled up on the floor of my husband's car and sobbed. It was a day without gratitude, and many more followed. I felt shame and embarrassment. *How could I let cancer happen?* I wondered how I could explain to my co-workers and patients that I had *cancer*. What if I met women I had tried to help, and they saw that I was now part of the cancer club? Wouldn't this show them I did not know what I was talking about? What would these women say to me? Shocked at my misfortune, I was fearful of my future. At that early point in my diagnosis, I was resigned to just getting through treatment. I had no vision of what lay ahead. I was too distraught to pray.

Many months later, as I reached the conclusion of my treatment, the thoughts in my head read like a news story summary: "Fifty-two-year-old female registered dietitian working in cancer care recently diagnosed with breast cancer, overweight, stressed, and in need of lifestyle changes." My emotions and thoughts were tangled up in my professional role and my personal shortcomings. Two years prior, I had completed my master's thesis, examining how weight gain increases the risk of breast cancer. I thought, *How ironic*. Now the questions were: Am I among this overweight and obese group? How did I, a dietitian, let cancer creep in? Did I cause my cancer? I *was* overweight, and I *had* let healthy habits slide for several years, but I was not ready to admit it. And I was not prepared to address it. It was too early, and I was immobilized with fear, confused about what my cancer diagnosis meant. Not long after that, I realized that I was no different from all the survivors I had helped.

My diagnosis in 2014 flashed light on areas that begged for change. During treatment, I reflected on what alterations to present habits I could embrace to move forward in a better frame of health. Well-versed about the risk factors for estrogen-positive breast cancer, I had a good idea of what this might entail, but I was not ready to begin.

Shortly after treatment was completed in 2015, my husband and I realized it was time to alter our lives for greater balance and joy. Over the next year, we sold our business and our home of the past twenty-one years in Connecticut and moved back home to Colorado. Reunited with family and friends, I healed physically and emotionally. The raw emotions and shock of my diagnosis faded. At the same time, I stepped away from my role as a cancer dietitian. These changes signaled the beginning of a new chapter, gave me great comfort, and started the healing process. I focused on rebuilding family ties and enjoying our home state.

After the treatments were complete, I spent the next two years dwelling in the space that includes follow-up appointments with doctors, mammograms, and learning my own "new normal." While practicing gratitude for support from my husband, children, and perfect strangers, I realized my emotions were a jumble of sadness, anger, and disappointment. Slowly, I was recuperating, but fear of a cancer recurrence rattled around in my mind and heart.

Fear Scuffs Away at Your Joy

Time heals many wounds, except for the fear of relapse. Not one survivor I have had the pleasure of working with ever tells me she is 100 percent certain that cancer will never come back. I am not alone in stating that no matter the number of years out from your diagnosis, a fear of a recurrence is in your heart and mind.

Like a pebble in our shoes, this fear, left to rattle around, will rub a raw spot. In 2016, two years after my diagnosis, that fear became a stone in my boots. I knew the risk of recurrence was greater with my extra pounds and declining physical activity. It was high time to address my increasing weight and return to greater amounts of movement. To begin, I returned to walking greater distances and lifting weights to strengthen my body. Scrutiny of my food choices revealed my love of sweets, which I indulged in while I healed. At the same time, I found a part-time cancer dietitian position. Ready to tackle my weight and eager to get back into the clinic, I began to appreciate the courage and moxie I had shown in getting through treatment and moving across the country. A new path emerged, and as I followed it, my jumbled emotions unraveled, rejuvenating my career. This new route was not solely for my benefit; I was going to use it for the betterment of others. For the next five years, I forged a trail to guide my work in the cancer center. A new mission was growing in me: an ambition to assist other breast cancer survivors. Fear had scuffed away at my happiness, and with that, fresh eyes and ears revealed the broader suffering of others like me.

Now I see that life after cancer treatment does not mean there is suddenly an end to physical and emotional pain. Financial struggles, lingering lymphedema and neuropathy, fatigue, weight gain, anxiety, and depression are some of the ways through which cancer steals life's delight. Treatment bills pile up while lymphedema prevents walking the dog or tossing a ball. Fatigue, a constant companion, hinders social gatherings. Anxiety and depression, the most common of thieves, steal happiness from your days, robbing you of pleasure in the simple things. And then, you are visited by fear of recurrence, stealing your joy at every turn.

First, I was witness to the joy-stealing thieves of cancer; then I met the thieves myself. What I saw in myself was the opportunity to do something about the scrapes and scratches that cancer leaves while robbing you of a healthier future. And then, I asked myself how I might alter the frame through which you see yourself. By changing the view of your cancer experience from a lens of bewilderment, what might happen if you appreciated the *triumph* you displayed during treatment? Having gotten through something really challenging, you grew a thicker skin, sought out help, and pushed through discomfort and fear. You soon realize you possess a superpower: *resiliency*.

Bending but Not Breaking

Indeed, resiliency is your superpower. Nothing can steal your joy unless you give it permission. Your triumph over treatments has prepared you for the next step. And although cancer thieves will appear now and then, the automatic pilot of life before cancer is off, which means you are preparing for the rest of your life. You have cast off your comfort zones by emotionally flexing and bending for weeks, months, or a year during treatment. Been there, done that.

You and I adore the sweet words "no evidence of disease," or *NED*, rolling off the tongue of the oncologist. Each time you are calmed by a clean mammogram, your doctor's reassuring words, or a milestone, the fear of relapse is lessened. Two years have passed by cancer-free. Another year and you are cancer-free. Gradually, a discovery appears: you have cast off the painful emotions of cancer diagnosis and treatment. You look back and see what you have done. Triumph over beastly breast cancer. You bent and swayed in the storm but did not break.

All of us have a story or two about bending but not breaking during our cancer treatment. Maybe yours includes days of nausea preventing you from attending events, or tender, painful radiated skin that kept you from working in the garden, but this did not destroy you. The stormy clouds of cancer treatment may have dampened your spirits, but you expanded your tolerance and patience while enduring the pain and discomfort of side effects. You are more resilient than you realize.

We build up our resiliency while in our teens when we make the entry into womanhood. As we begin to menstruate and are taught to clean our bodies, endure cramps, and tolerate the monthly inconvenience, we develop resiliency. As women, we acquire mental elasticity from a young age, honed by the ability to withstand menstruation and later, childbirth. Well-outfitted with this superpower early on, a clash with breast cancer intensifies it.

It took a lot of toughness to await your diagnosis then get through treatments such as surgery, chemotherapy, and radiation. A well-honed courage emerged to face down the side effects, as did humility to allow others to care for your family while you were indisposed. During treatment, you were required to shift away from a comfort zone and into uncharted territory in which you had little control. You were unable to settle into autopilot while you prepared for the next treatment and managed side effects. Rather than staying stuck, you can use these newfound skills in your survivorship years.

Cancer Takes Your Life Away, and Gives It Back

Although cancer temporarily filched my happiness, I realize now I was granted insights I lacked prior to my diagnosis. Previously, my approach to working with breast cancer survivors was one of haste and impatience. Giving nutritional guidance, recommendations for weight loss, and evidence of low-fat, low-carb eating styles dominated my interactions. Professionally, my comfort zone in life before cancer, or LBC as I refer to it, included ears deaf to the emotional impact that breast cancer has on women. After cancer, my new habit was to listen more and speak less—while infusing survivors with nutritional knowledge, of course, but more importantly, showing them their own direction toward robust health. I had let go of the restraints that cancer had placed on my physical, emotional, and mental capabilities. Cancer took plenty from me, and that included a rushed approach while meeting with survivors in my LBC. From cancer, I took back not just a desire to resume my career but my ability to listen with an open mind and a generous heart.

On the one hand, cancer takes your life away, and on the other, it gives it back.

For the next five years, I devoted myself to appreciating the compelling stories of survivors. Stephanie, a forty-five-year-old mother of two teenage children, endured unrelenting side effects; her treatments stripped her of the strength she needed to care for her family, do her work, and interact with her church community. Persistent reactions to chemotherapy seemed insurmountable, and while my nutritional skills were key to preserving her nutritional status, they did not preserve her happiness. Relinquishing her daily duties to others—her family, co-workers, and friends who became her lifeline—kept her health and family function intact. Stephanie bent in directions she did not know she could, but with her strong faith and a willing heart, she approached the end of her treatment not as a conclusion but as a beginning. First, she displayed her gratitude for her top-notch doctors and those who cared for her. Then, she made a commitment to pay this forward. Weaving her strong faith into her resiliency story, she now comforts and encourages others as they receive treatment.

Another survivor, Maya, a sixty-two-year-old woman, received seemingly endless chemotherapy treatments and lost sensation in her hands. Numerous nutrition visits involved reminding and educating her about keeping her strength up with plenty of calories and protein. Truly, her irrepressible spirit glowed while she showed me photos of her family and their lives. Maya recognized that while cancer had taken away sensations in her hands, it also gave her the blessing of having her daughter by her side to figure out what to feed her; without her daughter, Maya doubted she could continue treatment. As a professional seamstress, Maya was no longer able to sew due to numbness in her hands. Not one to back down or give up, Maya found a seamstress to replace her while turning her sewing and crafting skills into a business that makes products that other survivors use to make life more manageable during treatment and beyond. Both Stephanie and Maya maintained an attitude of gratitude, used their resiliency, and turned this into action for their own advantage and the benefit of others.

Cancer spotlights restrictions; it offers you the chance to address whatever has been holding you back. For me, this meant paying attention to the emotional side of cancer, not just nutritional guidance. I discovered that I was not limited to talking about what to eat to manage side effects. Instead, I leaned forward and inquired about what brought a survivor joy and who or what made them happy even when they felt awful. During my LBC, I spoke and listened with my dietitian brain; now I was using my emotional brain. In so doing, survivors and their families became more willing to follow my nutrition recommendations. Energized in a way I had not experienced before; I traded my habit of uninspired nutrition consultations for a message with genuine understanding and concern.

Your treatments highlighted whatever limits you placed on yourself at work or at home, or with your health prior to cancer. A voice in your head may try to keep the restrictions of your cancer experience. But with cancer disappearing in the rearview mirror, consider what happens when you prepare yourself to rediscover parts of your life that have taken a back seat, such as parenting, a much-loved career, and roles as a loving wife or partner, grandmother, or community leader. This is your chance to make a difference, build on a dream, or relish your life as never before.

Be Careful How You Talk to Yourself

Author Lisa M. Hayes penned a phrase advising you to be careful how you talk to yourself because you are listening. Regularly engaging in positive self-talk is powerful, as it sets expectations for better things ahead. According to numerous studies and many mental health experts, positive thinking leads to optimism. Recall the story about the study group that journaled about gratitude—they had more optimism for the future and fewer symptoms of illness than the group that did not focus on gratitude. Speaking to yourself about failure, mistakes, and frustrations not only makes you feel bad but also plants you firmly in an unhealthy place. These behaviors reflect stuckness, best known by negative messages going through your mind. You may have been baffled by the notion that you cannot go backward but cannot figure out how to get in gear to move forward, either.[8]

A big challenge among health care professionals like me involves how to best deliver health messages perceived as threatening to your self-worth. Pressed for time, doctors and dietitians want to inspire healthier habits as efficiently as possible while also seeking to preserve your dignity. A minor slip-up in the turn of a phrase, or a lack of empathy, can trigger a bristling response from the survivor. Not surprisingly, research offers techniques, such as the 5 A's—ask, advise, assess, assist, and arrange—that are shown to help medical professionals maintain efficiency while preserving survivors' self-esteem during difficult conversations.[9] In fact, health care professionals attend conferences and webinars to improve the delivery of difficult conversations. Another approach, often used by dietitians, is motivational interviewing, which focuses on understanding the survivor's concerns about habit changes and developing rapport around those issues.[10]

Briefly, think back to how you felt during a medical or nutrition visit. You may have felt yourself becoming defensive when the health care professional pointed out something you *know* to be true about your health; a nerve buzzes and you shut down. Trigger topics include weight, blood pressure, and recommendations to change eating habits. The dietitian must balance how she delivers the evidence-based information to diminish the defensiveness of the survivor.

Research from behavioral science experts suggests that one way to decrease the defensiveness to health messages and increase an openness to hear these messages is through a practice of positive self-talk or self-affirmation.[11] Repeating a self-affirming phrase, such as reminding yourself that the self-care example you set is the one your kids or grandkids will copy, makes you more receptive to health messages from your dietitian and doctor. Recited repeatedly, your self-affirming phrases increase the likelihood that you accept other nutrition or medical advice. You feel less threatened when the dietitian or doctor encourages a critical change. Positive self-talk moves you beyond past mistakes and generates momentum toward something far better.

Survivors are more open and more receptive to my message when they use positive self-talk to speak to themselves. They are also more receptive to me when they know that I am engaged and really listening. I knew when I heard a survivor tell me about her *gratitude* for her doctors, her family, and her perseverance and then list her plans for claiming her best life, she was spelling out the possibility for change. After these sessions, I could figure out how to take that self-affirmation and turn it toward what she wanted to change. It's easier for some survivors to do this, and it's not as simple for others.

Shedding light on how gratitude pulls survivors toward more positive thoughts soon became my first order of talking to a survivor. And introducing the concept of resiliency served as the springboard in maintaining momentum for new habits. I could bring it all together, joining nutrition education with new behaviors in a way far more powerful than nutritional guidance alone.

I also began to take heed while listening to those who expressed despair and hopelessness. Frustration and disgust peppered the words uttered by Jess, a sixty-year-old divorced mother of two grown daughters. Jess was among the first survivors who got the improved version of me. She sat down with me and gave me an account of things she had done "wrong" over her fifty-five years: too much sugar, no exercise, and fast food. She recited her list as though she had spent years in preparation for this confession. She gave me a sheet of paper with a hastily scratched note of her meals and snacks for the past three days. I sat quietly, waiting for her to tell me more. Instead, she glanced at me as if expecting a scolding followed by straightforward diet instruction.

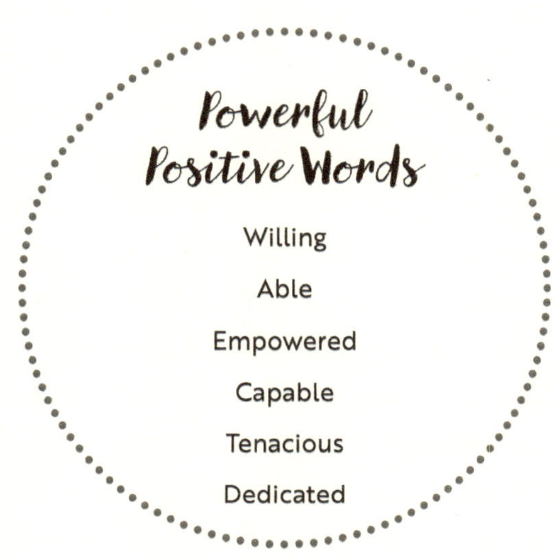

Instead, I began conversations with her about who and what in her life were giving her greater joy after her cancer. Her shoulders relaxed with my question, and her face softened as she told me how grateful she was for her daughters and how they were her inspiration for trying to get more physically active. With increasing energy, she further spoke of how she could do more with her daughters on weekends if she was more active during her workweek. Although she was not ready for momentous changes, this was a good place to start. Her gratitude for her daughters' love and attention quieted her despair and presented her with an invitation to talk to herself in a more positive tone. She saw a possibility in slowly increasing her physical activity during her lunch hour or after work, all because her conversations with herself were more hopeful and self-affirming.

In a word, Jess benefited from the opportunity to reflect on the value her daughters added to her life. Ultimately, Jess needed a softer touch delivered with an offer to reflect on the appreciation she felt for her daughters and to further examine current positive activities. Jess desired a prescription for gentle self-talk, not a grandiose meal plan or a finger-wagging rant about eating out too much.

The Power of Optimism

Related to positive self-talk is *optimism*, a cheerful outlook for the present and future, and *mastery*, which is the ability to cope effectively with daily challenges. Research by mental health experts shows that, combined, optimism and mastery are necessary for a positive outlook of the future. Positive thinking does not automatically appear after a cancer diagnosis. You may have found ways to spur yourself along with encouraging words, but many survivors have poor emotional health, anxiety, and lack of adjustment.

There is power in practicing optimism. Survivors who have hopefulness and an understanding of what they need to do for their health have reduced anxiety, better coping skills, and greater physical well-being.[12]

Importantly, breast cancer survivors who engage in self-help activities have less stress, perhaps because they feel that they have some control over their cancer. When I think about optimistic survivors, I recall that their successes came largely because they had positive expectations for their future. With what I call "knack," which is the same as what psychologists call self-efficacy, they felt that they could be successful in their efforts. Changes such as getting adequate sleep, increasing physical activity, and a healthier eating style—all self-help activities—are more readily adopted with optimism and mastery.

Optimism may not come easily to you, but speaking to yourself with greater admiration is a good place to begin. Practice talking gently to yourself. Like an attitude of gratitude, hopefulness begins with awareness and gradually becomes a way of thinking. Positive conversations encourage and reassure us that what we believed to be impossible *is* possible. The following box gives examples of positive self-affirmative phrases that you can practice. You can make up some of your own phrases using the list of Powerful Positive Words. You know yourself better than anyone else, so your own words are best.

An attitude of gratitude flexes the muscles of mental strength, which leads to resiliency, resulting in more positive self-talk while unleashing optimism. All this finally results in the mastery of new health habits. It adds up to a big *yes, you can do this!*

Self-Affirming Phrases

I am a good example of motivation and
confidence for my son and daughter.

My success at weight loss is related to how I plan out my meals daily.

I have all that I need within me, and I ask for help when I need it.

My family and friends support me and want me to succeed.

I am committed to doing what is right for my health; this
gives me the willpower to say no to sugar and alcohol.

Walk toward Your Why and You'll Find Your Way

Following our values is popularly known today as "walking toward the why." Other terms used to describe your why or purpose are intention, aim, plan, target, meaning, objective, and goal. Walking toward the why is crucial if we are going to stay on track with our goals. Consider instances when you have been influenced by someone with habits that go against your target to eat more healthfully. Perhaps you wanted to imitate their way of disregarding how unhealthy it is to drink sugary sodas at each meal, so you adopt a similar habit and add soda pop to several of your meals. Or maybe your family declares that holiday meals taste best with plenty of fat and sugar bringing maximum flavor, so you comply and bring a dish that suits them. Called "social contagion," behaviors and attitudes spread through crowds of people wanting to fit into what the crowd deems acceptable. When you lose your why, you lose your way. When you are caught up in social contagion, your resolve to create a new habit or shed an old one is threatened. With a strong sense of purpose and a defined reason for changing your behavior, your plans are not so readily hijacked by what everyone else chooses to do.

While all of this sounds newfangled, the concept of finding your why is not a new idea. During the Second World War, Viktor Frankl wrote about his experiences in Nazi Germany concentration camps, and he often quoted this phrase by Friedrich Nietzsche: "He who has a *why* to live for can bear almost any how."[13]

Your why does not come from a book or a good movie. Purposefulness is shown in the quality and focus of your actions. What does a walk toward the why look like? It is on display when a breast cancer survivor says she wants to be a role model of good health for her daughters and lays out a plan to teach them how to eat well. Determination to stick to a plan is revealed when a survivor chooses to reduce alcohol intake to decrease her chances of breast cancer coming back. A strong dedication to a goal is on display when a survivor goes on a four-mile walk each day so that she can hike with her brother and his kids this summer. When you keep your values in front of you, your options open; when you move away from these values, doors close. Our purpose and values begin in our minds and are fulfilled in daily actions.

To further understand this, think about eating out with friends, and someone at the table orders a generous portion of crispy, kettle-fried chips. The smell is heavenly, the browned rounds irresistible. Without thinking about your goal to eat more healthfully, you order your portion of these chips. What will it take for you to resist? Maybe while making your restaurant order, you recall how you wish to purposefully model for your daughters a healthier choice in foods. Or maybe a survivor recalls her reason for skipping dessert is to avoid a diagnosis of diabetes. All the willpower in the world will fail if you don't have a strong and purposeful motivation.

Of course, it is easy to get off course. Negative emotions and thoughts get in the way of your why. Damaging self-talk like "I'm not worth it," "I have never had good willpower," and "I always overeat at picnics" directs your mind and actions downward. As you learned earlier, affirmative self-talk reassures and encourages you to stick to your plan. Positive self-talk is proven to allow people with high-risk health habits, like eating too many kettle chips or avoiding a short walk at lunch, to hear positive health messages—even from their own lips. The nudge from a phrase such as "I know what eating too many kettle chips does to my cholesterol, so I will not order them tonight," spoken under your breath, may be enough to keep you (and me!) from going off track. Regularly practiced, positive self-talk helps you develop emotional agility. With greater ease, you move through thoughts of unworthiness as just passing notions instead of a backslide into previous habits. Having a purpose is the best path toward reaching our goals, but it will not magically appear. To discover it, you may have to dig deeper into what makes you excited to get out of bed each day and leave behind the things in your life that do not serve your purpose any longer.

My purpose did not jump off a page in a self-help book, nor did it come to me at the time of my diagnosis. Over time, a strong, health-driven desire to avoid a recurrence of cancer, along with the health issues of my parents, emerged. Next, my heart's desire was for time with my grown children and grandchildren, energy for traveling, and remaining fit enough to hike, fish, and ride horses, which became my social-driven purposes. Once I had these in order, I molded my habits to suit.

Examples of Health- and Social-Driven Purposes

1. **Health-driven purposes**: lowering cholesterol or high blood sugar, improving blood pressure, lowering the risk of cancer recurrence, decreasing joint pain.
2. **Social- or family-driven purposes**: hiking with grandchildren, adventure travel requiring walking, reaching work goals, looking good in clothes.

A sense of purpose can come from one or both categories. As you create your purpose or why, you will see if a combination of health and social purposes will drive you or if there is only one spurring you onward. Regardless, writing down your purpose for changing habits reveals that she who has her why to live well can bear nearly any how. Once your purpose is personal and real, behaviors change. Here are some purpose statement examples from other survivors:

- I want to slim down and attend my daughter's wedding looking and feeling great.
- I wish to strengthen my knees so that I can continue to walk with my husband every day.
- I want to avoid diabetes and all the problems with insulin that my dad had with the disease.
- I desire to control my heart problems and avoid another bout of breast cancer so I can be around for my daughter and son.
- I have travel plans that require me to walk two to three miles each day to see the sites.

The next chapter will go into more depth about health- and social-driven purposes and setting your purpose to drive you toward improved health habits.

> **Laurie's social-driven purpose for writing this book** stems from a desire to educate, inspire, and motivate fellow breast cancer survivors toward a healthier life using subtle and refined lifestyle changes.

Support from Other Survivors Is Life Support

My professional expertise, mixed with my value-driven purpose to help, moved me to conduct an experiment to see if I could be more impactful in driving and motivating my fellow breast cancer survivors to healthier lives. Plotting out my vision of what a program for breast cancer survivors could look like, I pieced together a course. I included assistance with weight management, cancer-fighting eating habits, and ways to get more activity. I paired a breast cancer survivors group with a nationally recognized weight management program. Over forty survivors participated in this hospital-based course, which lasted more than two years before gently closing with the onset of the pandemic. Participants first attended a ninety-minute education session I led to give them basic nutrition education about portion sizes, nutrition myths, calcium foods and supplements, and topics of direct importance to breast cancer survivors. Simultaneously, I reviewed breast cancer-specific nutrition facts as they attended weekly meetings. As time went on, something I had not planned for began to happen.

My course was intended to furnish targeted nutrition knowledge before participants began the weight-loss program, but something bigger was materializing. At their sessions together, each survivor was practicing gratitude and sharing a part of her experience that was personally meaningful. This was informal and unplanned, but weekly, they shared triumphs and setbacks, gave each other inspiration and tips, and allowed each other to offer self-forgiveness when one of them had a downfall. Then, they began to build and recognize their individual sense of purpose. Some of them would declare their purpose to bolster their motivation or show another member the value of their personal why in setting and reaching goals. Slowly, they built a toolbox of skills to improve their ability to adjust to slip-ups. Each passing week, I witnessed their increased confidence and optimism at staying on track and resetting any derailments. The group developed toughness as they navigated their failures or missteps. One with a setback would be put back on track by the others who shared their experience with getting through something similar. They built a powerful intention of confidence around their shared efforts to lose weight, find ways to move more, and eat foods that nourished and satisfied them. Their social contagion was positive. They found a way to satisfy their hunger to move healthy habits forward.

Some women in this program lost more than fifty pounds, and others increased their exercise/movement bouts to well over 150 minutes per week over the course of two years. During the isolation of the pandemic, some permanently lost track of their goals, proving to me that the support they gave each other was life support. Others kept some or most of their goals intact and continued to use the tools they had gained from each other despite no longer supporting each other face-to-face. Moreover, because some members of the group maintain their connections today, they continue to offer each other a safe place to receive a pardon, reset their goals, find another means of motivation, and gather their confidence.

I am a strong believer in the power of support we give one another. Of all the examples of cancer survivor triumph that I have had a role in, this group was the most meaningful. Reinforcing your life's goals within the chumminess of a support group of others going through these same challenges is that little extra that moves you up and over into healthful routines.

I want breast cancer survivors to become experts in their stories. I want to give survivors a shot at making lasting lifestyle changes, not flash-in-the-pan adjustments that only last a few short weeks. And I want these lifestyle changes to be administered with a lighter touch, one that moves you along gracefully and is sensitive to what you have endured. I believe in the power of gratefulness for those who got you through treatment, choosing hopefulness over despair, harnessing your proven resiliency for reaching your goals, and having optimistic conversations with yourself. Applied daily, these efforts keep the door wide open to positive changes.

KEY POINTS

- Enduring cancer treatment gives you a superpower: resiliency.

- Gratitude improves optimism about the future and reduces symptoms of physical illness.

- Positive self-talk moves you beyond past mistakes and generates momentum toward something far better.

- Walk toward your why and you will find your way.

- Support you get from other survivors is life support.

Trade Old Habits For Better Ones

"You can't reach for anything new when your hands are still full of yesterday's junk."

—ZIG ZIGLAR

BREAST CANCER SURVIVORS know that it takes one rogue, misbehaved cancer cell to wreak the havoc that initiates cancer again. The threat of a recurrence means survivors are rarely emotionally, physically, socially, and even financially free of the effects of cancer. Here in this spot of feeling trapped, a place of vulnerability, a *teachable moment* emerges. The teachable moment is a term popular among health educators who recognize it as the time someone is most ready to learn about a new topic or behavior. These moments can be linked to accidental events and unfortunate experiences, which cancer is. But a moment is far from sufficient for teaching better habits, never mind the time it takes to restore health. Survivorship could be better described as a teachable *era* because it extends for the rest of your life.

Your habits are not you, so you are not bad, but some of the habits you have are not good for your health. A tendency to skip yoga class, forget to drink enough water, or cave in to what the crowd is ordering for dinner are unfavorable habits, but these wayward leanings are not you. Rather, instances such as these are poor decisions, not your identity as a person.

For most survivors, life gets in the way of plans, and establishing better habits involves more than merely signing up for yoga, drinking eight glasses of water a day, or never giving in to what others are ordering around the table. No magic wand exists that will instantly create for you a new and improved habit. Real resolve is required to change routines. Besides, trading poor habits for better ones applies to all areas of our lives—including self-care, relationships, giving back, and better nutrition.

Embracing the opportunity to practice new habits for better health shows strength and perseverance. Substituting a better habit for a poor one implies creating a new comfort zone, one that shows triumph over not just cancer but the rest of your life. That is huge.

Trading old habits for new ones is an important way you take your life back from the clutches of cancer and from difficult social circumstances. Using a soft, feathery touch instead of a hammer to design your healthier future allows your confidence and capability to expand. In this chapter, you will:

- Assess your motivation, confidence, and viewpoints for tackling goals.
- Explore the details of putting new habits into action.
- Consider what situations stand in the way of new routines.

According to Nir Eyal, author of the 2019 book *Indistractable: How to Control Your Attention and Choose Your Life*, a *habit* is described as a behavior done with little or no thought, while a *routine* is a series of behaviors routinely repeated. Routines, Eyal says, are uncomfortable, and establishing a new one requires determined effort. Creating a routine of drinking eight cups of water daily or practicing balance while brushing your teeth requires patience, self-discipline, commitment, and a dedicated sense of purpose. And, after weeks or months of consistently drinking eight cups of water a day, a habit takes root in the daily rhythm of your life. Next thing you know, drinking more water is like your daily habit of tying your shoes.

Eyal believes that a behavior must be performed frequently as a routine before it can become a habit.[14] This partly explains why it is so difficult to acquire a new habit. I'll be using the words *routine* and *habit* interchangeably to reflect an understanding that first comes a new routine until, finally, a habit takes hold.

Old Habits Are Comfort Zones

A diagnosis of cancer often points to the failings of the body to keep healthy. Women with persistent routines of good self-care feel confused and betrayed. Daily exercise, a sensible diet, and managing stress—sometimes good habits are not foolproof insurance after all. How can my body allow cancer to grow? What did I do to cause this? Was it the stress of my job?

Others, after a lifetime of undesirable health habits, experience an "I told you so" self-defeating dialogue in their minds. A woman with harmful habits may claim it was only a matter of time until breast cancer reared its ugly head. A colleague of mine in the cancer clinic once confessed to me that she knew her risks for breast cancer were high; her family situation was chock-full of worry and regret. Roughly a year after her retirement, she was diagnosed with breast cancer; it saddened me to hear that her falsely-held beliefs about stressful family life and a breast cancer diagnosis had been fulfilled. In many instances, I have heard tales that women tell, admitting to a failure to take care of themselves and, as a result, getting what they deserve. Deserve cancer? No one deserves cancer.

A survivor making the remark that she caused or deserved breast cancer is saying she has not lived up to her expectations. But on the heels of the cancer experience, there is a chance to reset these expectations and create new ones.

Some women are hard on themselves. Our society sets high expectations of women, and some fall to the pressure while others shun it. Some are critical of their bodies, emotions, thoughts, and activities, which complicates how we grow and transform. Connections to others, notably your family and close friends, are important, and at times, our need to serve others takes priority over our personal wellness. You may analyze why you do the things you do, or you wonder how you can do better for others. Trying to figure out these behaviors and choices from a purely psychological approach may be too overwhelming and may require professional counseling. Some survivors may need this level of work to overcome beliefs, thoughts, and behaviors that prevent growth. Yet it is enough to claim that we think and do what we do because we are shaped by the patterns in our families and the social roles of our lives. For some, overcoming the obstacles that family life and social circles present is prickly. But it does not have to stay this way.

Recall for a moment the comfort zone of your old habits. Within the comfort zone is where you find routines, good and not-so-good. Family and friends have expectations that may involve placing their needs before your own. Maybe you are well-loved because of the way you remember birthdays, bring a special dish to dinner, and express kindness or sympathy when needed most. This comfort zone belongs to both you and your family/friend circle. Stepping out of this comfortable place and into the spot where you trade an old habit can be as simple as substituting for your prized cherry squares that everyone loves at the summer picnic with an arugula, pepper, and fennel salad. Or it could be letting your daughter know that you are putting aside thirty minutes each morning before breakfast for stretching and strengthening, and you ask that she please not bring the grandkids over until you are ready. Sure, people bristle at change and feelings get hurt, but you deserve the best for your health. By making small changes, you make progress on your goals.

Mickey, a survivor I spoke with at a regional women's event, shared with me that for years, she was a super-striver—community leader, professional, mother, wife, and carpool driver. Hyper-mode was her only mode, but most activities focused on the needs of others, not hers. In an unfortunate turn of events, Mickey was injured in a car accident, leaving her with a traumatic brain injury and unable to move or speak. During recovery from her brain injury, she was subsequently diagnosed with breast cancer. For anyone, this would be a double-whammy, but for this high-achieving woman, it was a wake-up call.

Due to her immobility and inability to speak, she had turned to food and soda pop as sources of contentment. But soon, her weight soared to over 250 pounds due to overeating and inactivity. After a long period of recuperation, she envisioned her way back to health, which meant tackling her burgeoning weight gain and debilitating state of immobility. Sensibly, she chose to apply a soft approach to decrease the daily habit of drinking several bottles of soda pop. Rather than drinking her daily allotment of sugary sodas, she made a goal to gradually cut them out entirely. Every day, she would drink several sips of the soda while saving the remainder for the coming days, repeating the same allotment of soda each day. Soon, she had stopped her daily soda habit. While this habit went unnoticed for weeks, finally her family took notice of the weight loss and how she was doing something for herself, taking charge of unfortunate circumstances to alter her health. This was the first signal, to herself and others, that she was changing course from super mom, professional, wife, and community leader and pivoting toward caring for herself first.

Modest changes, big impact. Quiet signals, change of direction. A little communication to signal your subtle changes leads to better acceptance among even the prickliest members of your clan. The great news is that once you have pushed against one family or social obligation and made a change for your good instead of someone else's, the next little change you make won't be as noticeable. With good communication and planning, contentment comes for both you and your friends and family.

Old habits are a comfortable place where you do not have to second-guess what you are doing, and nor does anyone else. But are these old habits giving you the life you have in mind for your future? Habits, good and bad, begin for a reason. Undesirable habits often spring out of stressful situations, helping you cope with family arguments by hosting the events yourself, avoiding physical activity so you don't inconvenience your grandkids' sched-ules, or keeping your friend from pouncing at lunch by agreeing with her restaurant choice. Stop trying to figure out why you started an undesired habit. Knowing why you formed this habit is not helpful. Your habits are not you. Your habits, good or bad, are who you are on autopilot.

There Is No One-Size-Fits-All Purpose

Brené Brown, a speaker and author of numerous books about vulnerability and walking toward your why, urges her audiences to reconsider the vulnerability that comes with a traumatic event, such as a cancer diagnosis, not as defeat or weakness but rather as an *opportunity* to sharpen commitment to our values.[15] A teachable moment is more than a favorable time to learn something; it is vulnerability speaking to you and inviting you to move in the direction of possibilities. This moment is a pause when you may hear the whispers of your purpose, your why, gently encouraging you to step forward. Just as you bent but did not break during treatment, you have what it takes to move you in the direction of positive changes. (Not yet certain? Practice positive self-talk for a few days and check back in with yourself. You may find you have a greater sense of purpose than you previously believed.) Survivors come with all sorts of dreams, nightmares, successes, and failures, and we have varied family situations and health concerns. There is no one-size-fits-all purpose for survivors, nor is there one goal that suits all of us. Perfect timing does not exist. Find *your* why and, at the same time, craft a goal or habit that suits your life's circumstances. You are not too young or too old, too healthy, or unhealthy, or too organized or messy to make goals for a healthier future. In "An Attitude of Gratitude," you were introduced to types of purposes. While there are other categories to describe your why or purpose, for this discussion about lifestyle changes, look toward two purposes: health-driven and social-driven.

Is Yours a Health-Driven Purpose?

News headlines, social media posts, magazines, and medical office brochures broadcast messages about decreasing the risk of cancer and other diseases with a change of health habits. In your life before cancer, you heard the advice but received no inspiration to act on it. In your life after cancer, these same messages prompt teachable moments.

Avoiding a recurrence of breast cancer is an example of a health-driven purpose. So is lowering blood pressure, preventing heart disease, or avoiding skin cancer. Lowering blood pressure implies a change in diet, medication, or physical activity. Avoiding skin cancer means more attention to sunscreen and wearing protective clothing when exposed to the sun. Health-driven purposes are tied to a change in daily schedules. A change in routines is tough, so the reason for adopting a new habit must align with your why; it must have substantial importance to you.

Early on in my dietetics career, while meeting with survivors receiving chemotherapy or radiation, I recognized that what I recommended required that you, the survivor, had to not only agree with my guidance but you also had to decide that nutrition was part of your cancer treatment plan. For the most part, survivors did this willingly and capably. Managing nutrition-impacted side effects during treatment implied selecting from a list of those foods that would not aggravate nausea or diarrhea, but this change to your daily routine was temporary. However, once treatment is completed and lifestyle changes for better overall health are desired, the approach swings toward making more permanent food choices. A sizable shift in planning, shopping, and preparing the food is required if you are to successfully follow the nutritional plan I have suggested. Your cooperation is required for the nutrition care plan to work.

Doctors prescribe chemo or radiation to treat your cancer, and you have little control over how much chemo or how many radiation treatments are administered. Your medical team figures out what treatment is needed to stop the cancer, and you comply by showing up for treatments. Changing habits for health reasons, though, is different than taking medication, receiving radiation, or having surgery. To take a medicine prescribed for high cholesterol or high blood pressure requires you to remember to take a pill or two each day. Health habits like moving more, eating less sugar or fat, and practicing balance require mindful attention every day.

Jokingly, survivors ask me if there is a pill they can take to provide the benefits of healthier habits or if I could simply wave a wand to sprinkle these changes over them for instant activation. Sadly, no, but as you will realize in later chapters, some habits have more potency than others, and still others are easier to activate. I propose behavioral changes, or food as medicine, but you decide whether to "take" the medicine. Behavior changes, which is what food as medicine entails, are harder to adopt than taking a pill.

Or Is It a Social-Driven Purpose?

Finding a health-driven purpose may come easier than establishing a socially driven one, and though both provide the momentum you need to change your habits, a social- or family-driven purpose may be more impactful. Recall from the previous chapter the discussion about finding your why to find your way. In a similar way, Frankl, the author of *Man's Search for Meaning,* suggests that when someone becomes aware of a responsibility to a person or a cause larger than themselves, that person is never able to throw away the meaning of their life.[16]

To illustrate, I share Sheri's story, which sticks in my memory. A sixty-year-old divorced woman, Sheri finished treatment around the time her mother moved in with her. Sheri had aggressive breast cancer that required surgery, many rounds of chemo, and radiation. Following treatment, Sheri gave little attention to her exhaustion and fatigue. A return to work was necessary to afford to keep her home. As a reflective and practical woman, Sheri considered how best to improve her health while caring for her mother. First, Sheri defined a socially driven purpose: her mother's care depended on Sheri's devotion and stamina. Next, Sheri devised her health-driven purpose: managing her stress and overall health for her own benefit and that of her mom.

The responsibility of caring for her elderly mother granted Sheri little time to devote to taking walks or going to the gym. Work and caregiver stress had increased Sheri's emotional eating episodes, and with a forty-pound weight gain, she knew she was at greater risk for breast cancer recurrence. To fit in a short walk daily, she reached out to her support network, asking for a friend to sit with her mother. We put together a list of lower-calorie foods for her to munch on when stress was off the charts, and we came up with positive self-talk phrases for her to focus on. Over months of getting more daily walks and addressing an undesirable emotional eating pattern, Sheri was calmer, had more stamina, and began to drop the unwanted pounds. And, because I believe in the power of support from others, I must mention that Sheri strengthened these changes in her habits with the support of other breast cancer survivors.

Sheri had both social- and health-driven purposes; you may have one or both. Her motivation to alter her daily routine was firmly planted in her determination to care for her mother with as little stress as possible and to lose unwanted pounds to reduce her chances of another bout of cancer or other illness. Once a breast cancer survivor recognizes the responsibility for another person or a project that is of importance to her, she finds the tools needed to meet her goal, no matter how tough. Likewise, once she recognizes that she can shed undesirable behaviors and stack small changes together to build better ones, she takes charge of her health in a powerful but manageable way.

There Is No Such Thing as a Wellness Garage

Looking for that quick fix, survivors ask: "What can I do to repair the damage caused by cancer treatment?" On the tail end of cancer treatment or even years afterward, you may see what is faulty in your body or life and frame these issues as if you are a broken-down car. You begin looking for a wellness garage where you can drive in for a repair and, a few hours later, emerge good as new. If only it were that simple.

One survivor's story stands out for me. Nadine came to me in search of mending a pattern of overeating, a habit she had held onto for years prior to her diagnosis of cancer. In her midforties and obese but otherwise healthy, she had three teenage kids, a full-time job in health care, and a supportive husband. Despite the blessings of her family, she was disgusted with herself. She could not understand why she had let this happen. With little time for self-care, she requested that I give her the solution to her overeating habits and overweight body. On the first visit, we talked about her purpose for wanting weight loss now and explored possible triggers for eating too much, especially after work. On the second visit, defensiveness, the kind you read about earlier, emerged after my recommendation to focus on more vegetables. Nadine became protective, shielded the overeating, refused the simplicity of first increasing vegetables, and presented her solution—a fad diet. She would lose weight quickly and, after doing so, adopt my increase-the-vegetables recommendation. She wanted a quick fix, as if her eating style could be dumped out like an auto technician dumps old oil during an oil change. But I discouraged the fad diet, reminding her of how this effort would be short-lived and ultimately not help her emotional eating episodes. Instead of hearing me out, she subsequently became more defensive, and that concluded our visits.

Altering your future health is not about driving your body, mind, and spirit into a garage and having it fixed and ready to return to life in a day. A process toward change should be more like strokes of a brush, soft and gentle. I wanted Nadine to see that she deserved a less drastic solution. If we feel broken, we first must acknowledge the work ahead as one of refinement, starting with an honest conversation with ourselves about past mistakes and future desires. Conversations such as the ones I had with Nadine proved to me that survivors have work to do—practicing gratitude, recognizing resiliency, talking positively to and about themselves, and envisioning a better future before embarking on an important lifestyle change. More than anything, Nadine needed reassurance of her value as a wife, mother, and co-worker. From there, she could craft a purposeful intention and begin the work toward habits to quiet her overeating episodes. Small tweaks: a feather, not a hammer.

Flexing the Muscles of Confidence and Motivation

A common scenario at the dietitian's or doctor's office goes something like this: You are educated about an eating style that aligns with managing high blood pressure. You get a list of foods high in added salt to limit, learn about the value of fruits and vegetables for lowering blood pressure, and schedule a follow-up visit. After the visit, you recognize that some of your food choices and frequent eating out do not align with a lower-salt eating style. Plainly, you see that there is room for improvement and understand the nutritional concepts discussed—plant-based eating, less dining out, plenty of vegetables, more salads, lower salt, and fewer processed foods—this makes sense. But as you arrive home, a sinking feeling in your belly whispers a lack of confidence for putting this new style of eating to work in your daily routines. Now feeling overwhelmed, you toss aside what you learned and wonder what comes next.

In fact, you had defined your health-driven purpose before the visit, and it was to get your blood pressure under good control with diet, and you felt motivated to do as instructed. But the sinking feeling in your gut says otherwise. What is missing? An assessment of your motivation and confidence. Simply put, you left the visit not knowing how to flex the muscles of self-assurance. Without confidence, you are not able to generate changes in your diet.

This scenario is common, and I have left out the important confidence evaluation more times than I want to admit. Health professionals make noble attempts to educate and even inspire survivors, only to discover that simple education and guidance are not enough. This is true, especially if it involves changing behaviors, routines, and habits. A breast cancer diagnosis often occurs as we approach our fifth or sixth decade, a period during which habits and routines are well-entrenched. Experience has taught me that survivors in their fifties, sixties, and seventies may believe it is too late to adopt new lifestyle habits. But adopting a new way of preparing, choosing, and eating is a challenge at any time of life. The truth is that the benefits of trading habits outweigh the aggravation of leaving behind long-held routines. And just because you are of a mature age does not mean you need not consider better habits because it is never too late to look forward to a healthier future.

Numerous techniques, tools, and approaches to improve a survivor's confidence and ability to build better habits have been studied. Some work better than others to resolve low motivation and confidence.[17] Woven into a desire to make a switch to more cancer-fighting foods, for example, are the stages of change that we all go through when grabbing on to better routines.

As an example, a dietitian or other health professional may ask you why you decided that now is the time to consider a lifestyle change. The professional may use a technique called the Stages of Change, which posits that people move through six stages when adopting a new routine or considering a pivot away from one thing and toward another. First, you begin to think about a change, what it might look like, and how it might feel; this is pre-contemplation. Then comes contemplation, where you consider how you might go about making the change. Preparation, the third stage, is when you begin to consider how, for example, you will fit in a twenty-minute walk after lunch. Next is an action stage, when you have begun to actively practice a new routine.

Two more stages follow—one is maintenance, where you troubleshoot how to keep doing your twenty-minute walk when other commitments get in the way, and the last is the relapse stage when a routine is interrupted by conflicting events, boredom, or declining motivation. Seeing how confident or motivated you are to implement these changes helps you avoid frustration. An unwillingness to take a daily walk after work may mean that you are in the stage of pre-contemplation and that you are not yet ready to actively engage in a regularly scheduled walk. Conversely, you may discover that you are further along in the stages of changes, an action stage, and you find yourself more than ready to not only walk daily but to go further distances each day.

Knowing where you are in these stages can guide the goals you set and steer your course toward achievable and manageable lifestyle changes. A similar but more readily applied method is the use of a tool called Ready, Willing, and Able, which shows you how prepared you are for making alterations.

Ready, Willing and Able

Ready: Am I ready to prioritize a change in my daily routine over other events and activities?

Willing: How important is the change to me? Am I willing to sacrifice something else to embrace this change?

Able: What is my level of confidence in my ability to make the change I want? Or do I need to acquire more skills or knowledge?

Are You Ready, Willing, and Able?

The Ready, Willing, and Able method first looks at readiness, as in asking if your daily life is ready for a shift in behaviors. Does having responsibility for a loved one pose too much difficulty to add another thing or activity to your list? How important is the change in relation to the responsibilities you carry? It may look like an argument in your head that says, "Is working on better balance of sufficient importance to me that I will skip morning coffee with my friends and instead attend a balance class at the local recreation center?" Finally, are you able to alter your behaviors? Is your fitness level advanced enough to attend a dance aerobics class?

Deciding if you are ready, willing, and able is an honest evaluation of where you are at a given moment. I found this technique useful for survivors approaching the end of treatment or soon thereafter. Often, after exploring what is entailed in a change right on the heels of treatment, they realize their fatigue levels show them the body is not yet able, although the mind is eager to begin. A survivor needs a high degree of all three—ready, willing, and able—to have the best success. However, survivors with low readings in the three categories can undertake a modest change, such as the one that Mickey chose when she incrementally decreased her soda intake. While you may not have all three factors in your favor to tackle a big lifestyle project, you can successfully take on a minor one. Repeat the assessment in the weeks, months, and years after cancer treatment to enlighten you as to where you are.

Other methods used to identify confidence and motivation and to assess readiness, willingness, and ability are techniques centered around goal setting, action planning, and motivational interviewing. Each of these techniques, although slightly different in approach, is effective in identifying low readiness or motivation, but these methods do not explain *why* a survivor is not motivated or how to increase readiness or motivation. Health professionals often use a looking-forward activity for this instead.

Your Two Futures

By reaching into the future, you can shine a much-needed light on the benefits of your choices. Let's use the example of a survivor named Sandy, who is attending her yearly visit with her primary care doctor. For several years, her blood pressure had crept upward, and her doctor prescribed medication. She took this for a while but did not feel any different, so she stopped. Her doctor also recommended a twenty-pound weight loss and a diet proven to help with high blood pressure, called the Dietary Approaches to Stop Hypertension eating plan. A referral was made to a dietitian, but Sandy never made an appointment. Her doctor led her through the Two Futures discussion.

They talk about making no changes to medication and diet. Sandy recalls the troubles her mother had after years of high blood pressure that resulted in a stroke, causing blindness and related dementia. Her mother had refused, for many years, to take her blood pressure medication. Sandy envisions her life and health five years from now. What does this health look like? Sandy did not take the medication, nor did she lose any weight or change her eating choices. In the future, her health will look like her mother's current health. Three grown children and four grandchildren are what get her out of bed each day. They give purpose to her days, with day trips each summer and overnights at her house in the winter. If she declines treatment and chooses not to alter her eating habits, she will probably end up much like her mother. And she may not be able to share in the lives of her grown children and grandchildren in the ways she loves most.

Two Futures

FUTURE 1	FUTURE 2
Make **NO** Changes to my diet, activity. Picture Yourself 5 years from now … and ask yourself these questions	Make Changes for a healthier habit. Picture Yourself 5 years from now … and ask yourself these questions
What does your health look like? What concerns do you have since you did not make any changes to your habits? What health problems do you have? Did you live according to yur sense of purpose by not changing your habits? How does it make you feel?	What does your health look like? How do you see yourself in this future? What health problems do you have? What health problems did you avoid? Did you live according to your sense of purpose by changing to a healthy habit? How do the changes you made fit with your sense of purpose?

However, if Sandy chooses to take medication and change her eating patterns, the future looks a lot different. Five years from now, she sees that her blood pressure is lower, and she is looking forward to taking her now-teenaged grandchildren on a summer vacation at the beach. Five years later, she is cancer-free, her blood pressure is under control, and her risk for a stroke is much lower. In choosing to take blood pressure medication and make important changes, Sandy has lived with the intention of delighting in her children and grandchildren with vacations and family events.

Looking toward examples of your Two Futures helps you recognize what is most important to you, what you want most from your life, and how what you do to take care of yourself lines up with your values and purpose. The beauty of this technique is that you can use it for difficult decisions—fitting in your daily walk, taking a stress-free vacation every year, or downsizing your home—the uses are wide open.

Important decisions require considering the positives and negatives of doing things differently. Just as buying a new house demands a closer look at the lower cost of your current home in comparison to a new one with a higher price tag, lifestyle changes require you to consider what happens if you choose *not* to make changes to your health habits. There is a cost in not making changes; remember what I said about stuckness? You cannot move forward when you hold onto the past. The Two Futures method of decision-making shows that when you cling to current choices and activities, you decline the chance to move forward. From my standpoint, a look at Two Futures takes away the defensiveness that survivors have during conversations with health professionals about the damage of "bad" habits. It is more appealing to explore the "what ifs" of better choices than to get stuck on feeling bad about an old habit that no longer supports your health.

Creating Lasting Habits

Survivors are not any different than people without cancer: all of us want instant fixes to our health issues. In recent years, with the rise in popularity of fad regimens such as South Beach Diet, keto, macrobiotic, Atkins, paleo, intermittent fasting, and raw diets, and the fast weight loss associated with them, survivors ask if these diets are a good choice for weight loss. One broad appeal of a restrictive diet is that the temptation of choosing from foods for which there is a human weakness, like sweets and starchy foods, is removed; all you do is eat from the diet list. No food decisions are needed, and while you can stick to a restrictive plan for a while, this soon grows tiresome because our bodies and minds crave a variety of tastes and textures. Fad diets are characterized by extremes such as food restrictions, costly supplements or products, controlled eating times, and a lack of scientific evidence, and they lack nutritional balance. Low intakes of important nutrients, as directed by a restrictive plan, can lead to muscle and bone loss, as well as a loss of energy for activities. Complicated, difficult behaviors like complying with the short list of foods from which to choose and time restrictions for meals are not doable for the long haul. In the end, restrictive diets seldom become an automatic practice for dieters, which is why many people fall off the wagon after a short time. As with any permanent routine, establishing a lifelong calorie-restrictive but nutritionally balanced eating plan takes time and planning. There will be more about calorie restriction coupled with nutritional suitability in a later chapter.

You and I know that building durable, lasting habits takes determination and persistence, and still, there is a popular desire for faster results. A quick internet search for "creating new habits" yields more than fifty entries, with many referring to how long it takes to form a habit. A team of researchers led by Phillippa Lally found that it takes somewhere between eighteen and 254 days, with the average being sixty-six days, to make a behavior a lasting habit.[18] Of course, as noted earlier, the more complicated the habit, the longer it takes to make a behavior automatic.

Recall that while your habits are done with little thought, as in on autopilot, routines involve a stack of behaviors regularly repeated. Some behaviors become habits more quickly. Results from several studies confirm that the more concentration required to perform a task, the longer it takes to make it a habit.[19] The same study by Lally also discovered that it took longer to make exercise behaviors into a habit than to create an eating or drinking routine. Think about that: while you eat three meals a day to provide your body with enough energy, physical activity is not a three-times-a-day occurrence. You must be more intentional and thoughtful about adding exercise behaviors or sticking to a short, restrictive list of foods.

If making exercise behaviors a habit is more challenging, then how many times must we practice the behavior before it becomes a habit? Years ago, it was believed that behaviors became habits if performed regularly, say twice per month or "frequently,"[20] but newer research has discredited this vague knowledge and demonstrated that it takes much longer than that, particularly when the habit is complicated. Importantly, research also states that efforts to create lasting habits may need continued support to help you perform the behavior long enough for it to become automatic. As a survivor, you have probably discovered this if you have tried to create new routines on your own. And once again, the significance of support from others—family, friends, a support group, and your medical team—cannot be dismissed.

With a team of reinforcements, your successes increase, and so will your confidence and motivation to continue. But what happens with interruptions to your habit-building? Travel plans, family reunions, illness, and other examples of life disruptions can derail your efforts. Research shows that missing a single instance of a new behavior will not lead you to a letdown. The day after you miss drinking your eight glasses of water may pose a challenge for getting back on track but will not lead to ultimate failure. Look toward the superpower of resiliency you acquired during treatment. You altered your life to accommodate medical appointments, changed food choices to manage side effects, and did all the little things you needed to do to keep going. Habit formation requires the sort of resiliency that asks you to acknowledge that life happens and there will be days when you are not able to follow your planned behavior to a tee. And that you will keep going, picking up where you left off.

Setting yourself up to adopt a new habit is critical for your long-term health. New habits help you thrive, not just survive. What can you do to ensure successful habit formation?

- Choose less complicated behaviors first.
- Acknowledge that creating a lasting, durable habit takes time.
- Anticipate interruptions and setbacks.
- Assign a trusted family member or friend to support your effort.

A simple defined behavior like adding fruit to breakfast and lunch will become a habit sooner than making over the entire meal. Adding short bursts of physical activity to your day becomes automatic more quickly than making a goal of thirty minutes of daily activity. Goals that are specific and doable, like a piece of fruit with breakfast and lunch, are more likely to be achieved. As time goes on, you add another habit of choosing whole wheat toast with breakfast and whole wheat pasta with dinner. Or you add five or six minutes to each activity bout until you reach a goal of thirty minutes a day. Gradually, one small change leads to another until you have achieved a much bigger goal—in this case, building an improved eating pattern and more physical movement. When you acknowledge that it takes time to adopt the habits that ultimately lead to greater health, persistence will emerge.

Shift your thinking to see that the gentle nudge to your daily habits creates a brighter picture of your future. Disruptions to your daily habit-building are minor compared to the major inconvenience and challenge of cancer treatment. You have within yourself all that is required. Give yourself the grace and kindness you need as you develop the habits you desire. Trading poor habits for better ones is a practice of steady progress, not perfection.

Strokes of Brilliance: Your Life's Canvas

Practicing a new habit takes more than a sloppily applied attempt at something new. Trading in old ways of doing things while adding new ones is a science, but there are also artful strokes of brilliance involved. Think about painting on a canvas; if you use a brush filled with too much paint, the strokes are out of line and thick, and while you add big pops of color, the result is a gummy, gloppy job. The same holds true for new routines. It takes time, patience, and positive, encouraging words to yourself, with an eye on the result: a healthier you. A smaller brush filled with just enough paint leads to a masterpiece.

The gentler touch with a smaller brush is an ideal way to describe how to apply lifestyle changes. But this is not what always occurs. It goes more like this: You sign up for a class or a program, excited to get back to feeling stronger and better. A week or two into the activity, you realize something is not right. While you believed you were ready to start yoga classes soon after completing radiation, you found out that your energy level was too low for sixty minutes of stretching, flexing, and holding. Or maybe you signed up for a cancer survivors' walking group, but the neuropathy in your feet prevents you from going as far as the others. These scenarios are not necessarily a bad thing because they give you the opportunity to apply your own stroke of ingenuity. You solve the issue of what you thought you could do versus the reality of what you can comfortably and safely do by adjusting the activity for the level you are at right now. Altering your plans to accommodate where you are strengthens the overall process involved in building a new habit.

It is better to begin with a miniature goal or even wait until your body, mind, and spirit are better balanced. You could choose to do twenty minutes of stretching exercises instead of a sixty-minute yoga class. Or you could opt to add minutes to your daily walks as your neuropathy allows or give water-walking class a try at your recreation center. Your perfection comes from beginning with a pocket-sized goal instead of a grand plan. For some, this means waiting until you have the proper amount of confidence and motivation to begin or until you are ready, willing, and able.

Lorraine, a sixty-two-year-old survivor who had completed treatment two years prior, was more than confident and motivated. Food-wise, she was practiced at getting enough daily protein, and her generous salad each day gave her confidence in her nutrition. She was ready to add more activity to her day and willing to do the work to improve leg strength so that with less leg pain, she could create the garden she loved. When we met, she had already decided it was time to address the dwindling strength that prevented her from gardening and other activities she enjoyed. After several visits with the physical therapist, she felt ready to branch out and do more. Since most of her friends attended Senior Strength class, she decided to do this for her fitness and the social support it offered. Her efforts were derailed soon after she began when her spouse was diagnosed with a serious illness. Life got in the way of her plans, and she needed to modify her chosen activity to devote time to taking care of her husband and attending medical visits with his doctor.

Sometimes it is best to modify the effort to a goal that fits better with daily life challenges. Lorraine decided that daily walks with a rotating list of friends who had flexible schedules to walk at varied times could replace the strength class until her husband was more stable. This allowed Lorraine to get an emotional boost from her friends and sustained her energy so she could give cheerful attention to her spouse. A stroke of resourceful thinking kept her on track to improving strength and stamina. Amazingly, she did not sacrifice what was important to her; she shifted her approach. She continued with her self-care and made accommodations for her husband's health needs.

Soft strokes artfully applied change the landscape of your healthy future, and like an artist adds color and dimension to accent her final work, light changes accumulate until one day, you notice you have new routines.

Resistance, People-Pleasing, and Sabotage, Oh My!

As a woman, you experience unique situations that arise when you put forth the energy to change habits. A disruption of deeply embedded habits causes a domino effect on those around you. There is a disturbance in the force, and you oversee that force. Culturally, women are consistently expected and pushed into the role of caregiver, tending to the needs of others. This poses unique conditions for forming new habits. As people-pleasers and nurturers, some women find it hard to focus on their needs. Some women will do whatever is necessary to maintain the status quo among family and friends. Doing what you have always done is easier than trading what was for what can be. Do you know why? Resistance. Resistance comes from those around you and from within you. The need to please others rather than take care of yourself is your resistance. Preferring the nice comments that others say about you instead of setting the expectation that you need some time for yourself is resistance. Spending more time on yourself implies spending less on others and forgoing the satisfaction of caring for others.

Resistance may go undetected initially. First, resistance is a raised eyebrow from friends as they witness you making different decisions about activities, drinks, or foods. Then, as your behavior becomes more consistent, questions and concerns emerge. An example of this comes from one of my experiences with alcohol. In the past, I enjoyed a daily glass of wine or a beer with my spouse or friends. But this habit has implications for my health, and I often decline or set a defined amount that I will drink. People around me often insist I join in, and some will pour me a drink even though I politely beg off. As I stand my ground, I eschew my pleasant, compliant demeanor. My pushback is an affront to the role I long filled of going along, playing nice, and pleasing others.

Breaking away from old habits is hard enough if you believe you are the only actor in the game of push and pull. Opposition from others certainly compounds the difficulty of overcoming sluggishness, but there is yet another force to be reckoned with as you adopt a new habit: your brain.

Neuroscience studies show that resistance is more than a word battle or a physical standoff among your social circle; resistance is hard-wired in the brain.[21] Your habits and behaviors, done repeatedly over time, form deeply grooved pathways. These deep grooves wire your brain so that you perform the same tasks in the same way, not only repeatedly but efficiently, carving shortcuts so the brain does not have to work as hard. These easier paths put up a fight each time you perform a new habit; the brain must work overtime to forge a new path. At times, resistance comes as a whisper, telling you it is time for your nine o'clock snack. Other times, it arrives as a gut punch, saying you will never stick to your after-dinner walk; you have never been successful at exercising, so why now? Resistance tells you to stay with what you are already doing; it is so much easier than attempting to change.

While a daily soda pop habit can easily be automatic, so can behaviors such as people-pleasing, prioritizing caretaking roles, and fitting in socially. The choice to stop drinking several cans of soda pop each day won't get you the same fierce reaction as presenting a new, healthier option for lunch with co-workers. Your pronouncement to co-workers has upset the lunchtime apple cart, but a decision to decrease soda pop can long go unnoticed because it only involves you. Sabotage comments may sound like this: "You were so much fun before you decided you weren't eating fast food anymore. Now I must spend more money on lunch." Recall earlier how Mickey chose first to cut back on her daily soda to address her weight gain. As time passed and she had success with this, she chose slight alterations to her eating habits. Her social circle fought back with sharp comments in the form of discouragement. There were probing questions concerning her approach to decreasing her food intake. A nutrition professional instructed her that following a vegan diet was her only option for accomplishing what she had set out to do. Undeterred, she cast aside each of these arrows of resistance. She began to live unapologetically for her own health. Standing firm by this principle, she discovered a new superpower: by taking care of herself, she could still serve others.

Defy the urge to maintain the comfort zone where you please others before yourself. Perhaps you were taught not to draw too much attention to your needs. But you got through cancer with loads of attention to your needs, and it was okay. Choosing to ignore the voice of resistance takes resolve and a determined focus. Sometimes you must step back to go forward, beginning with gratitude so you can make sense of your past, bring peace for today, and create your vision for tomorrow. You are trading old, worn-out habits for shiny ones. Your hands are free of yesterday's junk. You are moving on.

KEY POINTS

- Define who or what gives you purpose for creating lasting health habits (your why).

- Compare your Two Futures, one with and another without a change in habits, to demonstrate the future impact on your health.

- Adopt a simple habit that takes less time than taking on a complicated one.

- Overcome sluggishness and social resistance to new routines by demanding a firm resolve to take care of yourself first.

Food As Medicine

"Let thy food be thy medicine, and medicine be thy food. Life is short, the art long.
Wherever the art of medicine is loved,
there is also a love of humanity."

—HIPPOCRATES

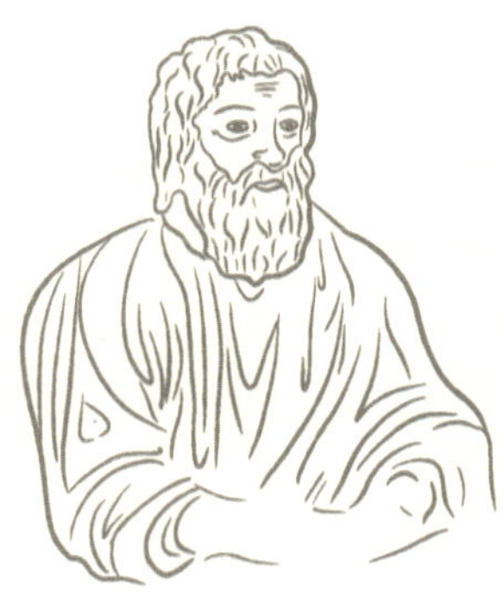

HIPPOCRATES WAS A GREEK DOCTOR living in 400 BC. He lacked access to nutrition and health research but understood the art and science of eating well throughout one's lifespan. Hippocrates may have been thinking about the anti-inflammatory diet, also known as a plant-based diet, when he referred to "food be thy medicine."

As a dietitian, I often take for granted what is familiar to me: food as medicine. You may not be as confident. Look at any women's health magazine today, and you will read about the anti-inflammatory diet, touted to prevent disease, boost energy, and improve health. These articles promote a means to improved health by introducing the basics about inflammation, but details about how to create the anti-inflammatory diet on your own are missing. I am going to provide them here and in chapter 4, "Puzzle Pieces," and chapter 6, "In the Pink."

The truth is, the anti-inflammatory diet describes *a collection* of eating patterns that embrace a focus on plant-based meals and snacks with less animal protein; less refined, processed, and added sugars; fewer processed starchy foods; more whole grains; a greater emphasis on abundant fruits and vegetables; a variety of oils for optimal health; and limited alcohol.

Anti-inflammatory eating patterns include the Mediterranean diet, American Heart Association diet, American Diabetes Association diet, Dietary Approaches to Stop Hypertension, and The New American Plate of the American Institute for Cancer Research. All of these diets are versions of plant-based diets, and each of these eating patterns offers a well-suited diet for breast cancer survivors. When followed regularly, these eating patterns can lower the risk of cancer relapse and decrease heart disease and diabetes. In principle, these diets reduce inflammation. Food is your medicine, your medicine is food, and when you eat well, you display your love for your own good health.

Re-read the last sentence of Hippocrates' quote: "Wherever the art of medicine is loved, there is also a love of humanity." And that means loving and caring for yourself. Food as medicine is more than food and nutrition; it is a philosophy of self-care. As such, the habits you cast aside are as impactful as the routines you embrace.

In this chapter, you will:

- Discover how diseases are initiated by inflammatory processes.
- Recognize that some foods contribute to inflammation while others reduce inflammation.
- Observe eating styles that prevent or manage diseases and support the nutritional health of breast cancer survivors.

Diets Do Not Work; Eating Patterns Do

Experts have established that condensing nutrition guidance into a list of foods or a specific diet to fight diseases like cancer or diabetes is not effective. Nutrition scientists are increasingly certain that eating patterns are superior to diets. As a reflection of this greater understanding, registered dietitians are encouraged to abandon the word *diet* and use *eating patterns* to describe how we speak about a survivor's daily food choices. Diets imply restriction, while patterns or styles suggest variation and flexibility.

Most of us have been on a diet more than once, perhaps even one of the fad diets discussed in chapter 2, but could you stick with this diet for your entire life? Not likely. The notion of a diet implies that there are lists of foods to eat, with restrictions or even avoidance of some food groups. The word "diet" encapsulates the word "die," suggesting that your effort to sustain it expires due to boredom, extraordinary hunger, or fatigue. A diet is inflexible, narrow, and rigid.

Conversely, an *eating pattern* is more of a portrait of the combinations of foods and drinks you regularly consume over a span of years. A pattern of eating implies a variety of foods available with few restrictions for times of day or the purchase of specific supplements. Which way of eating do you prefer? A diet sustained for a few weeks, perhaps several months, leaving you tired and uninspired? Or do you prefer an eating style that excites the mouth with flavors and textures while delivering disease-fighting, body-sustaining nutrients?

Ultimately, your choice of diet or eating style influences your health. And while the roots of disease are planted early in life, when eating routines may include too many calories, too much fat and salt, and too few fruits, vegetables, and unprocessed grains, it is never too late to pull up the roots of poor diet patterns and plant new ones. A change in food choices can stop a disease from advancing or prevent another one from establishing itself. You can gradually replace poor habits with better patterns by deciding to make every bite count.

The Real Deal about Nutrition Studies

Hippocrates may have been the original nutrition doctor and scientist. Despite this early evidence of the importance of nutrition, among all the sciences, nutrition is the least developed. Yet it is the most popular with the public because, after all, we all must eat. Luckily, each new study moves nutrition knowledge one step closer for experts and novices alike to understand how what we eat prevents or fights illness.

Although this is not familiar to most people, food and nutrition studies are imperfect in their design. Unlike medication studies that draw a connection to treating a disease, nutrition studies cannot definitively link certain foods to causing or curing diseases. Why not? Think about what is involved.

To research a study question about whether broccoli cures disease would mean that a group of humans would eat generous amounts of broccoli for months or even years. Most of the study subjects would quit after a short time due to boredom and the repeated appearance of broccoli at mealtimes. Nutrition studies rely on having participants recall the foods they have eaten regularly over the last several months or even the past year. Food records, which are imperfect because humans do not accurately recall everything eaten during the day, are nonetheless embraced in food studies as a method to show connections to a disease or condition. Imperfect study methods such as these mean that it is nearly impossible to show how a food can cause or cure a disease.

Finally, while many nutritional or food sites appear official, a second glance may show them to be just a cloaked opportunity to market a product. For these reasons and others, nutrition studies are some of the most difficult from which to draw conclusions.

Phony Nutrition Claim Phrases

"Everyone needs this"
"Provides strong prevention"
"Proven to work"
"Dramatic results"
"Natural ingredients"
"Detoxifies and purifies"
"Revitalizes your body"
"Effortless success"
"Immediate improvement"
"Guaranteed to work"

And yet, you and I read a nutritional nugget from a study blowing up the media, and soon thereafter, an urge to latch on to this tidbit of information takes over our thoughts, actions, and conversation circles. Next thing you know, the media, food manufacturers, and special interests are working to bend the minds of consumers to buy certain foods, products, or supplements. Cancer survivors are vulnerable to these messages. We want to get well and be well. Often, we will do whatever it takes, including accepting information containing a mere morsel of truth. Nutrition communications are not always based on proof, but media news flashes are attractive and can sway food beliefs.

Beware advertisements and headlines promising how a supplement can prevent, cure, or treat a disease. Alluring statements that sound too good to be true or lists of good and bad foods associated with a product are red flags signaling faulty information. However, a survivor equipped with a clearer understanding of food as medicine, such as found in this book, is ahead of deceptive food advertising and questionable nutritional statements presented by food manufacturers and marketers. By reading food labels accurately, better-interpreting food and nutrition terminology, and putting food claims in perspective, you are outfitted with tools to outsmart what is presented in the media.

What Is Inflammation?

As a medical term, *inflammation* describes your body's response to an attack or insult that throws your immune system into overdrive. There are two types of inflammation: acute and chronic. *Acute inflammation* is a short-lived response to an injury or illness, such as when an injured area turns red, swells up, and hurts. Once healing begins, acute inflammation resolves. However, *chronic inflammation,* the kind of inflammation addressed here, lasts much longer and is triggered by chronic infections, physical inactivity, obesity, poor gut health, diet, social isolation, psychological stress, disturbed sleep, and exposure to tobacco smoking, chemicals, germs, radiation, or viruses. Chronic inflammation exploits the function of our immune system, which is partly housed neatly within our cells. With sustained harmful insults like obesity, unhealthy eating, and mental stress, the immune system remains on high alert, causing the accumulation of components that can initiate diseases like breast cancer, type 2 diabetes, and heart disease, as well as depression and gastrointestinal disorders.[22]

Research has shown that there are connections between obesity and breast cancer, heart disease, and diabetes.[23] And in fact, researchers have discovered that the accumulation of fat tissue, which stores up these inflammatory components, is a likely link between obesity and these three diseases. Accordingly, the greater the amount of fat tissue, the more inflammatory chemicals there are within the cells, leading to a greater likelihood of illness from disease. However, less body fat means fewer inflammatory chemicals available to cause the illness associated with chronic inflammation.

Additionally, there are intersecting points between breast cancer and heart disease stemming from risk factors such as age, tobacco use, eating patterns, obesity, and lack of physical activity. But breast cancer treatment, both chemotherapy and radiation to the left breast near the heart, also increases the risk of heart disease. Some chemotherapy drugs are known to cause damage to the heart, and a scattering of radiation beams may reach the heart during left-breast treatments. As for the link between breast cancer and diabetes, experts believe there are four factors: high blood sugar, high insulin levels, hormonal imbalances, and inflammation. These are separate diseases, but the inner workings of how your body breaks down, uses, and stores energy create a greater risk scenario for survivors of cancer. A similar idea holds true for disease-fighting elements like how robust the antioxidants housed in your cells are and how effective your cells are at getting rid of inflammatory compounds that build up. Together, these factors impact your risk for cancer, heart disease, and diabetes.

> ## What would a registered dietitian say?
>
> Evidence shows that a modest weight loss of **5–10 percent** lowers the risk of recurrence of breast cancer as well as decreases diabetes and heart disease. This fact demonstrates that you do not need to be at an ideal weight or lose 20 percent or more to improve overall health. Modest weight loss is effective and achievable.[24]

Importantly, research informs us how each of these diseases can be prevented or managed well with lifestyle changes, such as anti-inflammatory eating patterns. Efforts to prevent these three diseases may serve as a keystone for a health-driven purpose for survivors. Furthermore, by practicing new lifestyle habits, survivors also discover how physically and mentally empowered they become simply by making small changes. In a word, by viewing food as medicine or physical activity as a remedy against disease, they are employing what they can do to ensure health. With pleasure, I recall the faces of survivors who report back to me their satisfaction with new routines, leaving them not only physically but also mentally and spiritually inspired. Nothing too elaborate, just soft and feathery but significant lifestyle changes, leading the way to health.

The Anti-Inflammatory Eating Pattern

Food as medicine. Sounds simple, but it is not. Confusing messages about what food to eat and not eat and which diet will "cure" diseases are anything but simple. Many survivors have sat with me, seeking reassurance and definitiveness about food choices. Often, a visit begins with a provocative question: Which foods fight cancer best? Then, often follows a request for a reduced-calorie diet for weight loss, and then lastly, a meal plan to make it all easier. What you want is a straightforward way to simplify decisions about what to eat.

The truth is, there is not a single food that fights cancer. Your body needs a variety of nutrients to fight disease. I am not a fan of weight loss directions for all, nor do I have a one-size-fits-all meal plan. Passing out a basic information sheet and meal plan fails to instruct you about the fundamentals of the anti-inflammatory eating style. More importantly, giving you a plan made without your input is not a plan for success. The anti-inflammatory eating style provides a foundation to address frequently asked questions, such as:

- Which foods best support my health to fight cancer and other diseases?
- How do I stick to a reduced-calorie eating style without unbearable hunger and boredom?
- What do I need to know to select highly nutritious foods?
- How do I successfully create a meal plan all my own?

By the conclusion of this book, you will have the tools you need to create your own brand of an anti-inflammatory eating pattern. For now, let's explore how anti-inflammatory eating styles and a small amount of weight loss curb chronic inflammation.

Nutrition science confirms that an eating pattern high in antioxidants found in fruits, vegetables, whole grains, and healthy oils offers the body a formidable cell-level defense force against inflammatory chemicals. The machinery in our cells runs better and manages toxins, viruses, and other invaders best if fortified with foods included in the anti-inflammatory pattern. Current research clarifies that one food alone cannot fight cancer; rather, it suggests that improving eating patterns is one of the best ways to shut down chronic inflammation. Recent studies from the American Society of Clinical Oncology have demonstrated that cancer survivors who consume a balanced diet have a 65 percent lower risk of dying from cancer than survivors who eat a poor-quality diet. Further, the study suggests that more than focusing on any food group, cancer survivors should strive for an eating pattern rich in a variety of vegetables, fruits, whole grains, proteins, and dairy at recommended serving sizes for age, height, and weight.[25]

Keep It Simple-r Changes

As a group, more than 40 percent of women sixty years and older are obese, according to recent health and nutrition examination surveys.[26] You understand the risks posed with being overweight and that your current eating habits may not be as balanced and nutritionally sound as you would like. Good news: modest weight loss comes on the wings of a healthier eating approach. It is like a buy-one, get-one-free deal. Not instantly fulfilled like presenting a coupon but doable over a few months or a year. There are ways to avoid starving, strictly following a meal plan, or losing oodles of weight. These ways begin with shifting how you view what to change and to what degree changes will impact daily life. There are three "simple-r" things you can do:

1. **Improve the quality of your eating pattern by choosing lean proteins, higher fiber from whole grains, and fruits and vegetables.**
2. **Focus on foods that are high in nutrient-density to support the health of your cells. Limit energy-dense, high-calorie foods that deliver few nutrients.**
3. **The combination of 1 and 2 will result in a modest 5–10 percent weight loss and improved nutritional health, thus lowering your risk of disease.**

A high-quality eating pattern includes groups of foods in amounts scientifically known to prevent diseases and sustain a healthy body. This eating style focuses on foods that keep you full and satisfied longer, which leads to eating less and, in turn, results in weight loss. This style of eating keeps you satisfied because vegetables and fruits are mostly water, which, along with lean protein and fiber, tells the brain that the belly is full. The result is you eat less but feel gratified.

Food as medicine in action means focusing on your food-group needs with nutrient-dense foods and beverages and gracious self-care.

Dietary Guidelines for Americans: Make Every Bite Count

Resolving chronic inflammation does not occur overnight. A slow reversal of the effects of inflammation takes time and good planning. Certainly, a diet rich in anti-inflammatory elements is a key to this. Around since 1980, the Dietary Guidelines for Americans (DGA) were fashioned by the Surgeon General with an eye on improving the health of all Americans. Many Americans yawn when reading about the Dietary Guidelines, if they read them at all. The DGA are rewritten every five years based on what we Americans are eating and how healthy we are. They are constructed based on the most solid nutrition science available and connect the dots between nutrition and health. Interestingly, as I was designing this book, a prominent cancer nutrition researcher, dietitian, and colleague of mine, Maura Harrigan, encouraged me to base nutritional guidance for this book on the DGA. Always the clever one, Maura reminded me that the touchstones of the anti-inflammatory diet are obvious in the recent DGA (2020–2025) and, therefore, support the guidance offered in this book. Finally, after reviewing evidence-based studies regarding breast cancer nutrition and health, I prioritized seven food categories within the DGA as the basis for the In the Pink Plate Plan introduced in the final chapter.

A particular genius springs from the DGA: each edition is based on Americans' eating habits while pinning down which nutrients we are lacking, then subsequently building new and improved guidance to set the nation's nutritional health back on course. You are not so different than non-survivors in what you choose to eat and drink; it's just that superior nutrition is of great importance for your recovery from treatment and, ultimately, health and survival.

To illustrate, most Americans do not consume enough calcium, potassium, dietary fiber, and vitamin D. Low intakes of these nutrients are linked to health concerns for Americans, but for survivors, eating enough foods with these nutrients is of greater importance. Most survivors' eating styles fall short of calcium (dairy foods) for bones, potassium (vegetables and fruits) for nerve and muscle activity, dietary fiber (whole grains) for digestive system health, and vitamin D (fortified milk, egg yolks, and fatty fish) for bone and cell health. Calcium and vitamin D intakes boost bone density, which is particularly important when taking anti-estrogen aromatase inhibitors. Potassium boosts nerve and muscle activity that was diminished from cancer treatments. Fiber intake improves belly health by boosting the absorption of valuable nutrients and eliminating toxins.

"Make Every Bite Count," a promotional phrase for a recent DGA revision, is appropriate for survivors like you and me. Making every morsel, bite, spoonful, and chunk of food count suggests that you view the foods you eat as contributors to your health and bringing more than flavor, enjoyment, and energy. Making every food tidbit count matters at every stage of our lives—baby, child, teen, adult, or survivor. The foods we select distinguish whether we thrive or merely survive. Like a menu that offers a restaurant's meal options, the DGA functions as a starting point.

Just four overarching guidelines are presented in the most recent DGA. We will concentrate on the third and fourth guidelines, as these are essential for women with breast cancer. These two guidelines (*) will be the focus for building your eating style. The second guideline dealing with personal, cultural, and budget considerations will be touched upon later. The four Dietary Guidelines[27] are:

1. **Follow a healthy dietary pattern at every life stage.**
2. **Customize and enjoy nutrient-dense food and beverage choices to reflect personal preferences, cultural traditions, and budgetary considerations.**
3. **Focus on meeting food group needs with nutrient-dense foods and beverages and stay within calorie limits.***
4. **Limit energy-dense foods and beverages higher in added sugars, saturated fat, and sodium, and limit alcoholic beverages.***

Nutrient-Density Defined

Nutrient-dense foods are chock-full of anti-inflammatory components like antioxidants, phytochemicals, vitamins, and minerals, all of which give our cells the stuff needed to fight off cancer and other diseases. Packed with vitamins, minerals, lean protein, and complex carbohydrates (more on these in a bit), nutrient-dense foods afford your body high-quality fuel for optimal function and disease-fighting power. Foods high in nutrients should take most of the room in your bowl, on your plate, and in your hand. Examples of nutrient-dense foods are:

- whole wheat bread
- fruits and vegetables
- lean, low-fat, uncured meats
- fish
- low-fat milk, cheese, and yogurt
- eggs
- nuts

However, there is a cautionary tale connected to nutrient-dense foods. A nutrient-dense food does not always mean that it is also low in calories; meats and low-fat milk, nuts, cheese, and yogurt are *not necessarily the lowest in calories.* Cheese is a prime example of a nutrient-dense food, as it is rich in calcium and contains protein but is also high in fat and calories. Similarly, nuts have plenty of healthy fats and protein, but a portion size is about one-fourth cup, roughly a handful, and it is too easy to eat two or three times the correct portion size.

Sticking to portion sizes as noted on a Nutrition Facts label, like the one shown in the next chapter, is as important for nutrient-dense foods as it is for a candy bar or a dish of chocolate ice cream. (More on an easy method to track portion sizes in the next chapter, "Puzzle Pieces.")

Energy-Density Defined: Crinkly Packages

Energy-density, or calorie-density, is the amount of energy or calories in a particular weight of a food. A chocolate bar may be small and lightweight but is high in calories and, as such, a suitable example of an energy-dense food. *Energy-dense, processed, and junk foods* are high in saturated fat, added sugars, and calories, mostly with *few, if any, nutrients.* Typically, these foods are mass-produced packaged breakfast cereals, crackers, cookies, reconstituted meat products, instant noodles or rice mixes, and soft drinks or sodas. Years ago, in a nutrition class where I was speaking about eating too much junk food, a gentleman asked a clarifying question. "So do you mean foods contained in crinkly packages?" At first, I hesitated, not quite understanding the intent of his comment. Then it sank in. "Yes," I replied and realized the great wisdom that comes from this statement. I have used it often to demonstrate a simple way to identify energy-dense, processed foods.

This category of foods is confusing because some healthy foods are energy-dense *and* nutrient-dense. Nuts are an example of a food both energy- and nutrient-dense, as I've mentioned. A handful of pecans, walnuts, or cashews is high in calories but also rich in nutrients, like selenium and healthy forms of fats. Go one step further in the confusion of how foods can be both nutrient- and energy-dense by adding a chocolate or yogurt covering to these same nuts. While the nuts buried inside the scrumptious coating are nutrient-dense, the outer yummy coating, which is energy-dense, in a sense "cancels out" the nutritional value of this choice.

Ice cream covered in cherries or strawberries is another example of canceling out the nutritional worthiness of nutrient-dense berries with energy-dense ice cream. Ice cream contains some nutrition in the calcium from the milk and cream that are used to make it. And the fruit topping has nutritional merit, but this value is overridden by the high saturated fat and sugars in the ice cream. Healthy recipes for fruit-based desserts are prepared with lower fat and less sugar, which retains more of the nutritional significance of the fruits. Though it's impossible to eliminate all energy-dense foods from your life, prioritizing nutrient-dense foods over energy-dense foods results in better health.

Eating too many energy-dense and processed foods can result in cancer and cardiometabolic diseases, which include diabetes and heart diseases. Research increasingly suggests that these diseases often cluster together, with cancer and heart disease the most common grouping. Yet these three diseases are preventable and manageable with improved food choices and lifestyle routines.

A large European multinational study including over 250,000 partic-ipants, mostly women, demonstrated that among women who eat more ultra-processed foods, there is an increased risk of not just one disease, most often cancer, but of having two diseases at the same time, usually heart disease as the second disease.[28] Among the women participating in the study, those who consumed 34 percent of daily calories from ultra-pro-cessed foods, mostly from artificially- and sugar-sweetened drinks and processed animal products (hot dogs, jerky, cold cuts), had a higher risk of having several diseases. Although sauces, spreads, and condiments were also linked to greater risks, this was to a lesser degree. Interestingly, the research suggests several explanations about processed foods and the diseases, one being weight gain and obesity from these foods and another in how processed foods require less chewing time, thus delaying a signal of fullness in the belly, which leads to overeating. Additionally, the researchers present non-nutritional theories about how processed foods increase risks, including unfavorable eating patterns, food additives, and contaminants from packaging. Any of these three may impact gut health and hormonal pathways (inflammation).

Perhaps the crinkly package advice holds more weight than I first believed.

With consistent practice, these two simple changes of more nutrient-dense foods and fewer energy-dense foods result in an important third change, a 5–10 percent weight loss over the course of months or a year. (In "Puzzle Pieces," the next chapter, there are further insights into following these simple but significant changes.)

Go Big for Nutrient-Dense Foods

The third guideline, *focus on meeting food group needs with nutrient-dense foods and beverages, and stay within calorie limits,* contains the knowledge you need to better understand the complicated terms and to guide you toward using food as medicine. This guideline has made my profession both rewarding and tricky. Terms used by nutrition experts read like a foreign language. A big part of my profession is education about nutrition terms, and I love the chance to help a survivor better understand nutrition language. For example, I enjoy comparing unprocessed grains with processed grains, organic produce with conventionally grown produce, and demonstrating how to critically read a nutrition news story, selecting nutrient-dense foods and talking about crinkly packages.

Nutrient-dense foods—what are they? Nutrient-dense foods are defined as foods that provide vitamins, minerals, and other health-promoting components and have little added sugars, saturated fat, and sodium.

Choosing more unprocessed foods leads to higher intakes of nutrients that your body needs to take down inflammation levels. As a side benefit, this also means you stay within calorie limits.

An example of a nutrient-dense food is homemade vegetable soup, a lower-calorie soup. This soup has lean plant protein, vitamins, minerals, fiber, and phytochemicals that promote health with little, if any, added sugar, saturated fat, or added salt. A bonus of soups is that the water adds to our sense of fullness and offers better hydration too. A broccoli-walnut salad is high in sulforaphane (a powerful anti-cancer plant chemical), fiber, and omega-3 fatty acids and is lower in calories than a serving of fries or chips. A glass of low-fat milk is high in vitamin D and calcium, two nutrients that a bottle of soda pop sorely lacks. A handful of walnuts are high in calories, about 190 calories in a handful, but these little nuggets eaten on a road trip or on the hiking trail also provide alpha-linoleic acid, selenium, and instant energy. High in calories, yes; high in nutrients, yes. The key is managing serving size: a handful, not an eight-ounce dish.

Nutrition-Dense Foods

Vegetables and fruits—all colors
Whole grains
Seafood
Eggs
Beans, peas, and lentils
Unsalted nuts and seeds
Fat-free and low-fat dairy foods
Poultry and lean meats

Notice that in the prior examples, calories are certainly important but the quality of the calories is critical to properly fueling your body and supporting healthful function within the cells, muscles, organs, and bones. I recall years ago when a fad diet, the cabbage diet, was popular. This diet was extremely low in calories, and while rich in cruciferous plant chemicals from the cabbage, other nutrients were lacking. Another example is when a survivor embarks on a 1,400-calorie diet suggested by a friend or a magazine article with no thought about nutrient-dense foods compared to those that are energy-dense. In other words, she thinks she can eat 1,400 calories a day, and if desired, she can eat all those calories from cake and that will be okay. No kidding, this occurred with an encounter with a survivor who consumed her allotted number of calories in three chocolate bars a day. She met the calorie limit, yes, but not the goal of a nutrient-dense eating style.

Staying within calorie limits does not imply a scrupulous accounting of everything you eat, but it does mean selecting a variety of nutrient-dense foods over energy-dense foods. Chocolate bars are certainly delicious and oh-so-easy to eat three a day, but the lack of nutritional value means this plan is reckless.

Go Easy on the Energy-Dense Foods

The fourth dietary guideline, *limit foods and beverages higher in added sugars, saturated fat, and sodium, and limit alcoholic beverages*, is as important as increasing nutrient-density. The fun, extra foods add negligible nutritional value and, when overindulged, contribute to extra weight and obesity. But read the fine print. It says *limit, not eliminate*.

You know the old saying: All work and no play makes Jack a dull boy. An eating style you can stick to has a mixture of mostly "healthy" foods and a few fun foods, so you do not become a bored girl. Allowing fun, energy-dense foods, like a square or two of dark chocolate or a sliver of pie, can and should be a part of your eating plan. Anti-inflammatory eating styles work because there is a place for indulgence; without it, you become disgruntled with the plan and quit. Knowing how to weave food pleasures into your eating style takes finesse, and with practice, you can master this skill.

Why does this matter? Because sticking to any eating pattern requires occasional allowances for little pleasures. It is your habits of eating over months and years that influence weight and health, not what you eat over one weekend or during a holiday meal. If you emphasize nutrient-dense foods, a healthy body will flourish. Too many energy-dense foods give your body excess energy. The extra energy gets stored as fat. You gain weight when you overeat energy-dense foods on a consistent basis.

Energy-dense foods like ice cream, fries, candy, cake, pie, chips, crackers, beer, and wine are enjoyable, and although they do little to nourish your body, they have a way of cultivating your spirit. Briefly, foods like these spike your blood sugar, giving you an instant energy lift, but too soon, blood sugar levels drop and leave you sluggish. You need small amounts of them to continue to enjoy your life and memories made with little dietary splurges with family and friends. Use your resiliency to get back on track after an indulgent weekend or holiday celebration.

Balancing foods between nutrient- and energy-density is the key to applying food as medicine. You give your body a wide variety of nutrients, so give in to a treat now and then while still managing your weight. It comes down to how a calorie budget is spent. With the right mix of nutrients and a careful eye on the number of calories for function and activity, the survivor's body performs at top-notch levels. An infusion of fun foods helps you stay on track with nutrition-packed foods you eat most of the time.

> ## What would a registered dietitian say?
>
> Sugars added during food processing include sucrose, dextrose, table sugar, cane sugar, syrups, honey, and agave. They do not include naturally occurring sugars found in milk, fruits, and vegetables. For most Americans, added sugars come from sweetened beverages, baked goods, desserts, and sweets.

I highlight these concepts because as we age, staying at a stable weight and losing a little weight are worthy pursuits, but as I have stressed, a greater willingness to alter a routine arises with a feathery, gentle touch, not the blow of a hammer. Restrictive, heavy-handed methods result in a brand of frustration pounding down success while leading to failure. I like this recommendation and favor a balanced, anti-inflammatory style to get there, albeit gradually. I like this nugget a lot because I know what you may be thinking: "I need to lose fifty, sixty, seventy pounds or more to be healthy."

Instead of focusing on extreme weight loss and deprivation, cast your gaze on using food as medicine, like a dietitian!

A Dietitian's Toolbox

Dietitians use tools to evaluate weight, not to be mean but to understand the health risks of a survivor; it is a starting point, not the destination.

For decades, dietitians have used the body mass index, also known as BMI, to see in which category our weight belongs. BMI is based on our weight in relation to our height. It is not 100 percent foolproof, nor does it tell the whole story about health, and it has fallen out of favor among medical professionals in recent years due to questions about accuracy and application to a diverse array of races, ethnicities, body types, and ages.

Should you wish to assess your BMI, you will find a link to a BMI tool available in the Resources for this chapter at the back of this book.

Where your weight is carried is more important than BMI alone. Waist-to-hip ratio or waist circumference are more accurate tools for determining risks for disease. Weight collected around your waistline increases your chances of having diabetes, heart disease, and other illnesses. Information on measuring waist circumference can be found in the Resources at the end of this book.

Using the waist-to-hip ratio, or waist circumference, as a snapshot of your health, a dietitian can begin the process of creating a nutrition care plan custom-tailored for you. Looking at the overall picture, the size of your waistline is an important corner piece of the puzzle of your overall health. Calorie calculations, which are the next step in creating your care plan, comprise a bigger part of the plan. In "Puzzle Pieces," you will review a demonstration of how dietitians create a nutrition care plan for survivors.

Calculating Calories: A Number Crunch

A calorie is the amount of heat energy required to raise the temperature of one milliliter of water, which is about one-quarter of a teaspoon, by one degree Celsius. Calories are how a dietitian determines the amount of energy needed to optimally sustain the functions of the body. I compare calories to a budget. Just like a household budget guides how much you spend on clothes, shoes, cars, or houses, a calorie budget directs the foods you choose to eat to stay within your calorie needs. And just as no two households have the same budget, not everyone has the same calorie budget because energy needs are affected by age, body composition, body size, climate, gender, hormones, temperature, and activity levels. Stimulants such as nicotine, alcohol, and caffeine can increase the rate of metabolism by as much as 15 percent.

A variety of tools, methods, and even machines can determine individual calorie needs, but most of these are used in hospitals, universities, and specialized health clinics. Most commonly, a dietitian uses mathematical calculations, some more complex than others, to estimate calorie needs for weight gain, loss, or maintenance. This numbers crunch is an educated guess about how many calories are needed. A trial period of several weeks or a month shows whether the number of calories is suitable. Too hungry? Adjust calories eaten daily upward by one hundred to two hundred. Gaining weight? Decrease calories eaten daily by two hundred to three hundred. Adjustments up or down are often necessary to bring about the desired weight gain, loss, or stability. A range of calories, for example, 1,400 to 1,500 rather than a defined amount like 1,463, is often supplied as a way of balancing out the guesswork involved in estimating calories. A range also considers that you do not eat the same kinds or amounts of food each day. Food intake varies by appetite, energy-density, and activity levels, to name a few factors.

Calculating your calorie needs estimate reveals some surprising information, particularly compared to the calories you currently consume. Survivors are sometimes flabbergasted when I show calculated calorie needs that are far less than their usual calorie intake. As we age, calorie needs decline, and often, so do activity levels. Think about the aging athlete who continues to eat as she did while training and playing her favorite sport. Once this level of intense activity declines, so must calories if this athlete is to avoid a burgeoning waistline. In the Resources section of this book is a link to a tool that can calculate calories for weight gain, loss, and maintenance depending on age, sex, and physical activity levels. More complex, advanced calculations are also available via this link if you desire to delve deeper.

Calculating calories gives a dietitian the framework needed to build meal plans for you. You may have seen meal plans in women's magazines, on social media, or in an app on your phone. As important as the prescribed calorie range calculated are the foods included in the plan that manage or prevent disease and, very importantly, provide balance across the four food groups (more on those in the next chapter).

Counting calories or following a meal plan is instructive for most survivors in the short term, although a few embrace this level of regulation for longer. Accountability or responsibility to someone or something, like a dietitian, an app, or a logbook, is a good way to learn about mistakes, such as overestimating how much you've eaten. After you acquire a better understanding of food as medicine, learn to calculate calories, build a meal plan, and select foods for optimal nutrition, then daily calorie counting will subside. Over time, you'll become familiar with identifying calories and portion sizes, and a new habits will form. I have seen too many women become trapped by counting exact calories, only to become disenchanted and discouraged, then give up the effort of eating well altogether.

However, I heartily endorse a trial period of keeping track of calories as a method of informing you of how effective your estimated calorie budget is in helping you reach your goals. Even though eight weeks, or the sixty-six days it takes to create a new habit, may seem like a long time, the information you gather by doing so makes it easier to adjust your food intake up or down to better meet your needs. Another tool, perfecting portion sizes, is a smart way to help with calorie intake while instructing you on how it feels to stick to eating the estimated number of calories. Find more on simple ways to measure portions in the next chapter, "Puzzle Pieces."

Does Sugar Feed Cancer? Yes, And ...

Does sugar cause cancer? The minute a family member receives a cancer diagnosis, someone in the family begins an anxiety-driven internet search for answers to a suggested connection between sugar and cancer. This is among the most popular food-related questions posed among survivors and their families. Over the years of answering this question, the first words out of my mouth are something like, "Before quitting all sugar, it is important to better understand how sugar feeds cancer."

Over the years, I have recrafted my "Does sugar feed cancer?" explanation, but regardless of how I frame it, the answer is complicated. In a nutshell, this discussion centers around both *added sugars* and *processed starches.* Added sugars from soda pop, candies, jams, ice cream, and syrups, plus processed starches found in cake, pie, cookies, and many baked goods, are of greatest consequence for explaining the sugar and cancer connection.

Once broken down in the body, sugars and starches become glucose, the body's preferred source of energy for the muscles, heart, brain, and body organs. Sugar feeds every cell in the body, including cancer cells, and this form of energy is critical because it is also used to power organs and muscles. And because sugar is so important for your brain function and overall energy, your body will do whatever it takes to keep adequately fueled with it. For the remainder of this discussion, *glucose* will be referred to as *sugar.*

Research shows that the connection between sugar and cancer has to do with high insulin levels.[29] Insulin is a hormone and a chemical with the important job of binding to receptors that open the channels to allow sugar into the cells. During normal cell function, insulin efficiently signals the opening of these channels, and sugars pour in. Abnormal cell function, such as happens with inflammation, appears when insulin does not latch on to receptors, channels remain closed, and sugar is not allowed into the cells. This results in excess sugars, now freely circulating in the body, and if shut out of the cells, this extra sugar is stored as fat and further creates *insulin-like growth factors.* The combination of too much sugar floating around, the storage of fat, and these growth factors can initiate cancer cell growth, which is a prime example of an inflammatory process in the body. Other growth factors add to cancer cell growth, too, but insulin plays a major role.

Now imagine an eating style full of added sugars and processed starches. This eating style lacks nutrient-dense foods like fruits and vegetables, whole grains, low-fat milk and cheese, fish, and lean meat. An energy-dense, high-sugar, and processed-starches eating style is an ideal setup for cancer cell growth and inflammation. Too much sugar and not enough nutrients is an inflammatory style of eating.

Truly, you begin to recognize that just eating sugar does not necessarily fuel cancer; rather, the connection stems from eating too many foods with added sugar and white, processed starches that often lead to weight gain. One more concept to understand is that extra weight accumulated around the midsection of your body can alter the effectiveness of insulin, which is known as *insulin resistance*. When the cells in your body do not respond well to insulin and cannot use glucose for energy, the pancreas makes more insulin, resulting in a rise in glucose levels. So, the way in which sugar feeds cancer is a cycle. Too much sugar results in the storage of body fat and, in turn, leads to a condition of insulin resistance and, finally, elevated glucose. Sugar does not directly feed cancer, but it feeds a process that leads to excess fat, which contains inflammatory chemicals that can spur cancer growth.

Sugary foods and drinks, along with processed starches, make up the junk foods category, and admit it, total elimination is not a sustainable reality. Fixating on how sugar feeds cancer frequently leads to the avoidance of all sugars and starches, both good and bad. By doing so, fruits, whole grain breads and cereals, milk, and yogurt—all nutrient-dense foods—are purged along with candy and cookies. Limiting, not eliminating, added sugars and processed starches tamps down inflammatory chemicals and directs insulin correctly while helping cells function properly. A discerning approach to balancing nutrient- and energy-dense foods results in satisfaction rather than disgruntlement with your eating style.

All or None: The Problem with Quitting All Carbohydrates

"None, nothing, not even one, not one
mouthful of carbohydrate shall enter."

The temptation to quit all carbohydrates, added sugars, processed starches, and complex or "good" carbohydrates is driven by the fear that sugar feeds cancer. Giving in to this impulse leads to a disastrous result. Applying food as medicine means that the habits you choose to do away with are as significant as the new ones you adopt. Just as eating too much sugar leads to inflammation and disease, eliminating high-fiber, nutrient-dense complex carbohydrates leads to nutritional calamity.

Digging a little deeper, we learn that a *complex carbohydrate*, first defined in 1938, is a polysaccharide (poly=many, saccharide=starch or cellulose) made up of a chain of thousands of monosaccharide units (mono=one). Rice and pasta are complex carbohydrates, as are bread and breakfast cereals. Beans are made up of complex carbohydrates and protein.

As an example of what happens when complex carbohydrates are deleted, consider the gut's response to a lack of fiber from whole wheat bread or pinto beans, both complex carbohydrate foods. Fiber from brown rice and whole wheat pasta plays a role in maintaining bowel movement regularity, and without fiber from these foods, the gut slows and constipation occurs. Additionally, vitamins such as thiamine, B6, riboflavin, niacin, biotin, and folate are found in whole grains, cereals, and a variety of fruits and vegetables. Vital nutrients such as these are critical for the optimal function of many bodily processes. Choosing to avoid complex carbohydrates eventually results in vitamin deficiencies impacting brain and nerve health, the breakdown of foods in the gut, and the health of red blood cells. Minerals such as phosphorus, cobalt, manganese, iron, and selenium are critical for cell, muscle, dental, gut, blood, and bone health and are found in complex carbohydrates such as grains, beans, and leafy greens. Plant chemicals found in fruits and vegetables act as antioxidants, responsible for ridding the cells of toxins and compounds that cause disease and illness. Cutting out all carbohydrates, sugars and complex carbohydrates alike, is not a realistic option for maintaining health.

Finally, some complex carbohydrates are more nutritionally valuable than others. Fiber from brown rice, whole wheat bread and pasta, whole grain cereals, leafy greens, and beans regulates gut health, makes you feel fuller longer, and helps you retain the vitamins and minerals in ways that processed carbohydrates—white bread, rice, and pasta, to name a few—do not. Stripped of important nutrients, the white versions of carbohydrates have nutrients but not in the same power-packed amounts as unprocessed rice, pasta, breads, and cereals. You can have it all while nourishing the body with much-needed vitamins, minerals, and plant chemicals without feeding cancer. Embracing all carbohydrates, mostly the good ones but also including a limited number of so-called bad simple sugars and processed starches, is a balanced approach.

News Flash: New Controversy about Saturated Fat and Heart Health

Added sugars, processed starches, and saturated fats go hand in glove. These three are frequently mixed together in snacks and fast foods. For many years, you have read media articles stating that eating patterns low in saturated fat are linked to lower LDL, or "lousy" cholesterol, and good heart health. Recently, though, there have been doubts, questions, and a pause: maybe saturated fats are not so bad after all. But not so fast, according to researchers, because while there are now questions about the strength of these older saturated fat recommendations, there is not enough information for experts to support newer guidance that would approve of more saturated fats in our eating patterns.

To clear up the confusion, the American Heart Association and other heart-health organizations delved deeper into the new reports and decided to continue to support a recommendation of eating no more than 5–6 percent of total calories from saturated fat. As an example, with a 1,500-calorie eating pattern, this means seventy-five to ninety calories from saturated fats, or roughly eight to ten grams, an amount that adds up quickly.[30] The current Dietary Guidelines for Americans takes a slightly different stance on saturated fats in that no upper limit of saturated fats is specified; rather, the focus is on the overall eating pattern and not a recording of how many grams of saturated fats are eaten each day. Generally, a safe approach to saturated fats is to replace them with polyunsaturated fats, such as olive or avocado oils. Further discussions about saturated fats appear in "Puzzle Pieces," "In the Pink," and "A Brighter Shade of Pink."

Americans tend to prefer combination foods, which are usually made up of carbohydrates, protein, and saturated fat. Examples of combination foods include:

- tacos and burritos
- pizza
- cheeseburgers and sandwiches
- macaroni and cheese and casseroles

Whole foods that are high in saturated fats include:

- lamb
- beef
- pork
- poultry, especially with skin
- beef fat (tallow)
- lard and cream
- whole milk
- butter
- cheese
- ice cream
- coconut (fresh, oil, milk)
- palm oil
- palm kernel oil

Other foods that are often high in saturated fats are desserts, candies, ice cream, and fried foods. In other words, energy-dense foods are higher in both fat, sugars, and processed starches. Overall, fun or "junk" foods high in fat and sugar should comprise no more than 15 percent of your total daily calories. Ideally, the remaining 85 percent of total daily calories are derived from the four food groups—fruits and vegetables, whole grains, milk and dairy, and protein foods (beans, meats, fish, eggs). In the next chapter, "Puzzle Pieces," you will learn more about how these concepts fit into your nutrition plans.

Rather than counting grams or calories from saturated fat, focus on the overall quality of your eating style and read the Nutrition Facts label, such as the one found in "Puzzle Pieces," to find saturated fats in foods. Turn your attention to eating foods made with healthier oils, like olive, avocado, walnut, and canola oils, and avoid tropical oils, such as coconut and palm oil, or butter, which are very high in saturated fat. Incorporate fish and nuts into your pattern. Replace some meat with beans or legumes. Substitute pumpkin puree for some of the cheese in mac and cheese. Switch to healthier polyunsaturated and monounsaturated fats, which you will learn more about in chapter 6, "In the Pink." These changes, although simple, go a long way to lower your intake of saturated fat.

Become a "Less Than One and Done" Alcohol Snob

Survivors are surprised when I introduce drinking alcohol into nutrition consultations. Some survivors view alcohol as nothing more than a means to a relaxing end of a day with only a passing thought about the impact it has on health. What does alcohol have to do with food and nutrition? Despite the splash of orange or cranberry juice and a twist of lime, consider that beverages with alcohol are energy-dense with scant nutritional benefit. And although you cannot alter a genetic tendency to have cancer, nor can you change your age, you can choose whether you drink alcohol and, if so, how much. Study surveys conducted by the National Cancer Institute show that most Americans are not aware that alcohol causes several types of cancer, including breast cancer.[31] According to the World Health Organization, nearly 4 percent of cancers diagnosed worldwide in 2020 were related to alcohol consumption.[32] Among those who are aware, there's a belief that the risk of causing cancer varies by the type of alcohol. For example, more participants supposed that the cancer risks from alcohol were from hard liquor and beer, while some held to the belief that wine lowers your cancer risk. Hundreds of breast cancer survivors and I have discussed this, negotiated, and even cried over this.

Martina, a fifty-something survivor of early-stage breast cancer, had heard of the risks of alcohol and a recurrence of her breast cancer, but that did not prevent her from bargaining with me about the two-beers-a-day ritual on her back porch after her workday. Talking through tears, she eventually agreed to switch to non-alcoholic beer. Months later, I spoke with Martina, and she had adopted the non-alcoholic beer begrudgingly, but she appreciated her own determination to do the right thing for her health.

In the end, these discussions about alcohol and other unhealthy habits are not about your doctor or dietitian; the decisions you make about your habits are yours alone. The recommendations are made to assist in educating and guiding your decisions, not in making them for you. Beer, wine, and spirits are connected to socializing, relaxing, and savoring the fine things in our lives. But alcohol is not a nutrient-dense food, and it adds empty and extra calories, too. No one wants to admit to the downsides of alcohol. But alcohol and breast cancer do not mix well. Binge drinking, defined for women as more than four drinks in a single setting, may also add to breast cancer risk and relapse. Even drinking low levels of alcohol (less than one drink a day) carries an increased risk of breast cancer. A large study of women with early-stage breast cancer (postmenopausal) showed that survivors who drink three or more drinks weekly increase their risk for recurrence or death from breast cancer compared to women who did not drink alcohol. And this may be particularly true for postmenopausal women who are also overweight.[33]

Alcoholic drinks contain ethanol, which is a known carcinogen, and there are several ways researchers believe it may cause cancer. You have probably read about the heart-healthy properties of red wine and assume that wine, red or white, is beneficial for your health. The truth is that the ethanol in all alcoholic drinks, and in both red and white wine, beer, and spirits, can increase estrogen in the body, which increases the risk of breast cancer. The breakdown of ethanol in the body can also create high levels of acetaldehyde, a chemical produced in this process, which damages DNA and prevents repair of the damage, which may lead to the development of breast, liver, head and neck, and esophageal cancers.[34] In recent years, the American Institute for Cancer Research has revised a recommendation to read that no amount of alcohol is safe for breast cancer survivors.[35]

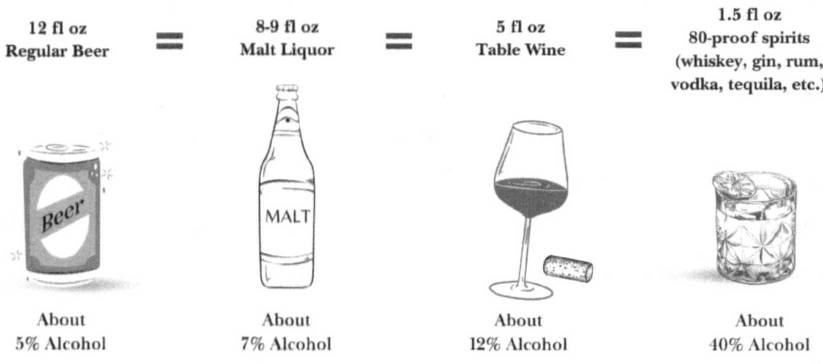

The percent of "pure" alcohol, expressed here as alcohol by volume (alc/vol), varies by beverage.

Adapted from Rethinking Drinking, National Institutes of Health, accessed October 16, 2023, www.Rethinkingdrinking.niaa.nih.gov.

A serving of alcohol is twelve ounces of beer, five ounces of wine, or a 1.5-ounce shot of distilled spirits. Important note: craft beer varies widely in how much alcohol is in a twelve-ounce serving. Check the ABV (percent of alcohol by volume) on the labels. You could be drinking two alcohol servings in just one beer mug. Some argue that resveratrol, the plant component in red wine, is healthy for your heart, but resveratrol is also found in red grapes, red grape juice, peanuts, and dark chocolate. You don't need alcohol to get resveratrol!

Because alcohol intake is one of the few adjustable risk factors, educating the girls and women in your life about the links between breast cancer and alcohol affords you an impactful role in the health of others. As I have shared with the young women in my circle, drinking alcohol, particularly in heavy amounts (more than seven drinks per week), increases breast density, which, in turn, increases the risk for breast cancer.[36] Be an alcohol snob and stick to less than one alcohol drink per day, which suggests drinking less than the usual servings and not every day, to avoid breast cancer relapse or even death. You will be making a positive change to prevent cancer's return, act as a positive role model, and save calories for cancer-fighting foods.

It Is Never Too Late to Build Better Habits or Get to a Healthier Weight

The foods we eat are more than just flavors, taste, texture, energy, or nutrients. We connect food to family celebrations, emotional comfort, nourishment for illness, memories of love, and caring for others. An eating pattern that cherishes the memories, comfort, and celebration of food alongside the nourishment it offers is a perfect union. And it makes no difference if you are twenty-seven or seventy-seven years old or have years of bad habits behind you. It is never too late to begin practicing food as medicine and creating healthier habits.

Eating is not just a habit of counting calories or following a meal plan; it is a daily practice and one that should be done with the best intentions. Eating is social, emotional, and psychological. Ignoring these factors is a recipe for disaster. I favor small tweaks to eating styles that lead to improvement of eating style quality. Concentrating on nutrient-packed foods and

limiting energy-dense ones leads to a 5–10 percent weight loss when practiced over weeks, months, or years. This approach puts the emphasis on
improving the eating style and making every bite something you count,
not calories.

Change can be as complicated or simple as you want. Choices that you
reject or replace are as important as new habits you embrace; this is self-care.
Deciding to limit added sugar, processed starches, saturated fat, and alcohol
is a good place to cast off food choices with low nutritional value. In "Puzzle
Pieces," the next chapter, you will discover more about the food groups,
those building blocks you learned about as a child, and how to select foods
that lay the foundation for an improved eating style. While I do not believe
in superfoods, I do believe in developing another superpower in you—one
that recognizes the impact of putting the pieces together, one at a time, to
create the picture of optimal survivor health.

KEY POINTS

- Food as medicine is a philosophy of self-care; the habits you toss aside are as important as the new ones you adopt.

- Chronic inflammation and obesity are linked to breast cancer, heart disease, and diabetes.

- Diets do not work; anti-inflammatory eating patterns do.

- Focus on foods that are high in nutrient-density to support the health of your cells. Limit energy-dense, high-calorie foods offering few nutrients.

- It is never too late to begin to choose foods with more nutritional value.

CHAPTER 4
Puzzle Pieces

"Be patient. Everything is coming together"

—MILLIONS OF THERAPISTS AND MOMS AND
DADS AND SUPPORTIVE PEOPLE WORLD-
WIDE FOR EONS AND GENERATIONS.

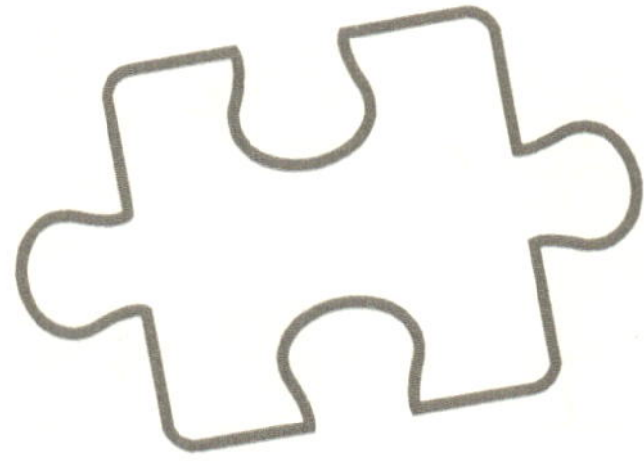

WORKING TOWARD A HEALTHIER LIFE is like putting together a puzzle. When you open the box, you are aware that you will not be able to complete it on the first attempt. With a thousand or more pieces, it is going to take several sittings. First you spread out and examine the pieces on the table to see which colors and patterns match up. Separating the straight-edge pieces first, you assemble the puzzle frame. Next, you match pieces of the puzzle that obviously fit together by colors and patterns, nudging them into place. The little success with easy pieces fitting snugly together moves you to keep going. As you continue working on the puzzle, you find pieces that you thought easily fit together but then discover they do not. You set them aside until later. You continue with the pieces, putting one corner together, then the middle section, until you have created a beautiful picture.

Putting your health back together after treatment looks like the pieces of a puzzle scattered on a table before you. You know the pieces go together, but it is not clear how or why. One piece at a time fits perfectly with another piece until the whole picture is revealed. This chapter builds on what you have discovered about adopting a "food as medicine" philosophy. This way of living poses questions such as:

- What are my health risks based on my body's current weight and shape?
- How much is the portion size of various foods?
- Of the four food groups, which one is the most significant for my health?

So, to begin putting the pieces of your nutrition puzzle together, this chapter will:

- Examine the roles weight and eating styles play in determining your risks for breast cancer recurrence, heart disease, and diabetes.
- Enhance your knowledge about how the four food groups interlock to form your food as medicine eating pattern.
- Review updated nutrition topics to nudge into your eating style.
- Show how a nutritional care plan is assembled for a survivor.

Resist the urge to rush to put the last piece of the puzzle in place; gradually, you will see what is needed to assemble the entire picture. The concepts presented here take time to understand and apply; some will be of little use to you right away, while others fit exactly with what you have already constructed.

Weight-y Things

I do not like talking about my weight or yours, but as a health professional, I know how body weight affects health. An increasing number of studies present considerable evidence that weight gain often occurs after a woman receives a diagnosis of breast cancer. Notably, numerous studies have reported that most breast cancer survivors experience weight gain, gaining somewhere between two and twelve pounds during treatment or in the five to ten years that follow. Reasons for weight gain include decreased physical activity and chemotherapy-related metabolic changes.[37] There are no clear answers about why weight gain occurs, but there are several dietitian-inspired thoughts on this.

During treatment, physical activity levels drop, which leads to a loss of muscle and poor exercise capability. If you had chemo with side effects, like nausea or gastrointestinal upset, your clinic staff advised you to eat processed and refined foods like saltines, gelatin, toast, canned fruit, cold cuts, soups, cereal, and ice pops. You may have continued with this eating habit beyond treatment and put on a few pounds as a result. Anti-hormonal drugs, like tamoxifen and aromatase inhibitors, while not proven to cause weight gain, alter our bodies in a way that either leads to weight gain, makes it hard to lose weight, or both. Furthermore, the onset of menopause, either brought about by these drugs or naturally occurring, changes our metabolism from an energy-burning one to a slower, more sluggish one. Unfortunately, the alteration in metabolism is stubbornly opposed to weight loss and favorable toward weight gain. Additionally, emotional eating sometimes creeps in. A more sedentary lifestyle during treatment leads to less muscle mass. All of this means that you cannot burn off extra calories as easily as before the diagnosis.

Two survivors, both with other health problems besides breast cancer and well into their seventies, demonstrated to me what it is like to tackle stubborn weight gain in more mature years. And yet, both women, Babs and Joan, were able to *maintain* their weight by improving the quality of their eating patterns. Holding weight steady is a victory in menopause. Another message I hear is that losing weight is too hard, especially after the challenge of treatment, followed by getting back to the rest of your life—family, work, and community. The difficulty seems colossal, particularly if you think a big weight loss is the only weight loss worth working toward. And only if it can be accomplished quickly. But minor tweaks to food habits, like adding more lean proteins, fruits, vegetables, and higher fiber foods, over time, lead to a modest weight loss. A reasonable weight loss like this improves our health, and more survivors are catching on to this information.

Not Gaining, Losing, or Maintaining? Try Tracking Portions

If you were to say to me that you are not gaining weight, not losing weight, or that you are not maintaining weight, the first thing I would ask is whether you are tracking and measuring portions. What helps is truthful and consistent measurement of the foods you eat. Carrying around measuring cups and food scales is not practical. You have what you need to measure portions right at your fingertips and in the palm of your hand. Measuring your food is tedious, but if you memorize the hand symbols for portions and read the labels, you increase your awareness of your calorie budget and meet your goals.

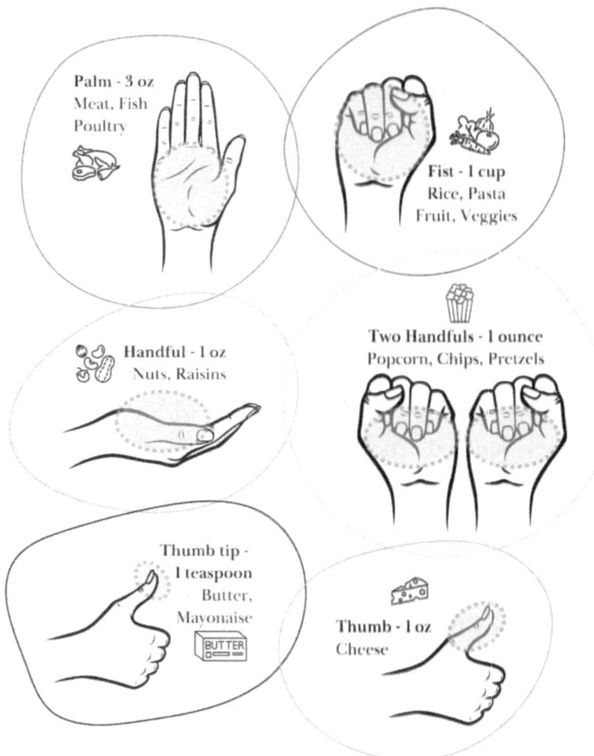

A portion of lasagna is the size of your fisted hand, which is about one cup. The thumb tip is a teaspoon of oil or sugar. An ounce of chips or pretzels is measured in two handfuls. Practice this handy way of measuring; commit it to memory.

Regular measurement of portions does two things: it makes you stop and examine the quantity you have on the plate, and it sets expectations for what you need nutritionally, not what you desire. Portion size knowledge fits well with reading a Nutrition Facts label. The label shown is for frozen lasagna, which contains four servings. As mentioned, one cup is a serving size, a fist-size, and in this serving, there are 280 calories. Moving to the area marked part 3, protein, carbohydrate, and fat contents are listed. Finally, and importantly, part 4 is a column listing percent daily value, which is a recommendation based on a two thousand calories daily diet as indicated in fine print at the bottom of the Nutrition Facts label.

Take a moment to look at fat and saturated fat. Notice that one serving of frozen lasagna provides 12 percent of the total amount of fat recommended daily and 23 percent of the recommended saturated fat. Outside the label are notes: 5 percent daily value is low; 20 percent or more is high. This lasagna is high in saturated fat because the daily value is more than 20 percent, which is considered unfavorable. Now go down to the part of the label where it is shown that the lasagna provides 25 percent of the recommended daily value for calcium. This is a high-calcium food, a good thing for bone health. As you read through nutrient discussions throughout this book, these terms will mean more to you and aid your selection of foods as you shop and prepare food.

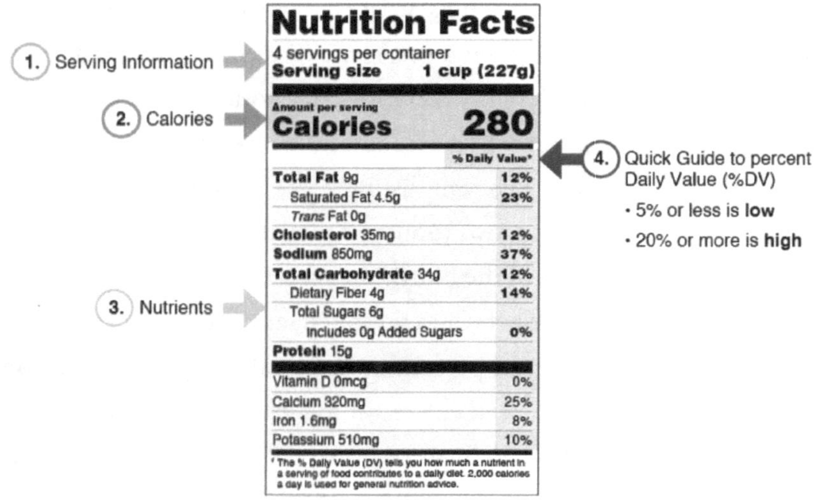

Nutrition facts label downloaded from the US Food and Drug Administration at www.fda.gov/food/food-labeling-nutrition/ nutrition-facts-label-images-download.

Cancer Care: Getting More Personal

More than 90 percent of us will survive breast cancer for at least five years. Similarly, 84 percent of women diagnosed with breast cancer will be alive after ten years.[38] Thanks to early detection and improved treatment methods, survivors are living longer and healthier lives. With diligent self-care, such as considering food as medicine, you can live a long, healthy life, but you should know about other risks and what you can do to prevent them.

Cancer treatments now pay more attention to other parts of our personal health, mostly due to a better understanding of how breast cancer, heart disease, and diabetes are related. Heart disease and diabetes do not affect all breast cancer survivors, but it is important for you to know the connections and how cancer treatment is changing to address them. Heart disease, not breast cancer, is the number one killer of women. In fact, treatments for breast cancer, both chemotherapy and radiation, put you at greater risk of heart disease. Chemotherapy drugs commonly used to treat breast cancer affect heart function. Radiation therapy, particularly for the left breast, also increases our risk of heart disease.

More hospitals are adding cardio-oncology clinics to address the health of the heart through cancer treatment and beyond.[39] Chemotherapy infusions are now given with the input of a heart doctor, who can help to guide the cancer doctor to give chemotherapy without damage to the heart. In radiation therapy clinics, doctors are directing attention to deliver radiation to the left breast with a barrier around the heart to protect it.

For years, cancer doctors have been aware of how diabetes and breast cancer impact care. Researchers believe that one likely connection between breast cancer and diabetes is weight gain, particularly for women who received chemotherapy. But another possible link is the steroids used to treat nausea and inflammation during chemotherapy, and they can lead to ongoing high blood sugar after treatment is completed.[40] Adjustments to treatment are made to help maintain blood glucose levels in a healthier range.

Over the past two to three decades, researchers have sought out how to reduce not only breast cancer recurrence but also diabetes and heart disease with improved eating patterns. Progress is being made, although it is slow, particularly as these experts work to discover stronger connections between these three diseases. One study conducted at Harvard found that a Diabetes Risk Reduction Diet (DRRD) may be an important lifestyle modification for breast cancer survivors.[41] Interestingly, the DRRD includes nine food categories commonly recommended to prevent diabetes, and they easily fall into place to support cancer and heart disease prevention too. Although further studies are needed to better understand how the DRRD or any another dietary pattern with a focus on nutrients and food items (notably coffee in the list that follows) may or may not contribute to calories, eating patterns like the DRRD are showing promise in how food choices impact the metabolic processes that promote breast cancer tumor growth. A recommendation for more coffee, decaffeinated or caffeinated, is from my viewpoint problematic, but this beverage has few calories (without the creamers) and contains anti-inflammatory components which may stifle diabetes, heart disease, and cancer. Appropriately, the list forms an eating pattern, not a diet, with words like "more," "less," "attention to," and "decreased" to suggest and guide, not advocate for nor push to eliminate certain foods. A list of the nine recommendations included with the DRRD:

- more cereal fiber
- more nuts
- more whole fruits
- more polyunsaturated (healthy) fats
- more coffee, caffeinated and decaffeinated
- less saturated and trans (unhealthy) fats
- attention to lower glycemic index foods
- decreased sugar-sweetened drinks
- less red meat

While it may not be apparent, your health after breast cancer has to do with you taking responsibility, and that implies careful consideration of how to fit all the pieces together. As learned previously, quelling inflammation with alterations in food choices and lifestyle habits decreases the risk of heart disease and diabetes, resulting in overall better outcomes for breast cancer survivors. In the big puzzle picture, this means you live healthier for longer. Gaining knowledge about four notable food groups is a good way to nudge pieces into place.

Fruits and Vegetables: Superstars of Cancer-Fighting Foods

You may have had a mother who nagged you to eat your fruits and vegetables. You may have grown up hearing that an apple a day keeps the doctor away. These sayings go through my head when I educate survivors on the importance of this food group, and though the phrases are outdated, I begin with fruits and vegetables because most of us do not get enough, and this group includes the superstars of cancer-fighting power. I am often asked which fruit or veggie a survivor should eat. Blueberries? Acai berries? Kale? My response is always the same: there is not one fruit or vegetable that is superior to the others. You need a variety of colors to get all the plant nutrients available to fight cancer and other diseases. This explains the popularity of the phrase "eat a rainbow of colors" of fruits and vegetables.

Most adults in the US do not eat a rainbow of the recommended five to seven daily servings of fruits and vegetables. My experience tells me that women do better at this than men, but regardless, two missed opportunities arise when you do not get enough: one is the chance to enhance health, and the other is personalizing culinary creations for ethnic and cultural enjoyment.

First, this food group outperforms the other food groups in the variety and density of the plant nutrients that help our bodies function optimally. And, while you may not realize it, plant nutrients contribute not only color but also flavor. Fruits and veggies are the superstars of nutrient-density and of fiber, texture, color, and taste. This food group makes all the other groups—meat, dairy, and grains—stand out and satisfy the palate. Fruits and vegetables are the edge pieces for your eating habit puzzle. They frame everything else that you eat.

Second, fruits and veggies allow you to customize meals to meet cultural, personal, and budget concerns. Thai food, for example, is recognizable by bamboo shoots, mushrooms, lime, onions, and chiles. The array of spices like mint, cilantro, ginger, coriander, and garlic tell my taste buds and my brain that I am eating Thai food. When I think of Italian food, I think about tomatoes, garlic, oregano, and onions. The vegetables and spices bring together the pasta, the meat or fish, and cheeses into the flavors and mouthfeel I crave. A little-discussed fact is that the human body best absorbs nutrients when several are combined. So, through the generous use of fruits and vegetables in many ethnic foods, your body is getting the benefit of numerous nutrients, each helping the others to be absorbed in the best way possible.

Fruits and Vegetables Detoxify

The word *detoxify* is everywhere these days. For our discussion, detoxification is a process occurring in the liver involving the cleanup and removal of bad compounds that are related to the development of diseases, including cancer. In a body well-fed with fruits and veggies, detoxification occurs regularly, like magic. Antioxidants in fruits and vegetables and whole grains are champion detoxifiers. They chase out bad compounds and clean up the resulting mess.

Antioxidants include carotene, flavonoids, sulforaphane, and many others. These superstars take the lead in helping cells to naturally detoxify and eliminate invaders from entering the body from food, medications, water, air, and even your own body processes. When these bad compounds break through our natural barriers, the body's detoxification system goes into superhero action. More details about the superhero abilities of antioxidants appear in chapter 6, "In the Pink."

Detoxification decreases the negative impacts of toxins, drugs, and environmental offenses. These bad compounds cause tissue damage, providing a starting point for cancer, heart disease, and diabetes.[42] And eating adequate fruits and vegetables daily gives your body enough antioxidants to clear out the bad compounds; with too few antioxidants available, the process occurs incompletely, and bad compounds are left over to do damage to cells and tissues. Plant foods, including unprocessed grain foods and fruits and vegetables, support detoxification all day long with abundant antioxidants.

Whole and Refined Grains: A History Lesson

For centuries, humans have eaten the harvested seeds of grasses, more well-known as grains. Rice in Asia, corn in Mexico, and wheat in the Middle East have served as staples of diets all over the world. In most diets, grains make up more than half of all the calories consumed. Grains are the staff of life for millions and are linked to reducing heart disease, diabetes, and some cancers. In recent years, grains have developed a soured reputation in the US, often billed as "poison" and the root of diseases. What happened to a food group that, years ago, represented bounty and health?

Processed foods.

Grain processing began in the 1880s because bakers and consumers requested a softer texture, longer shelf life, and improved taste for breads. The removal of the outer shell of wheat takes out fiber and lots of nutrients, leaving behind the inner portion, the endosperm, and a rich source of carbohydrates. The endosperm is the whitest, softest, and sweetest part of grains of wheat, corn, and rice. The remaining part of the grain makes up most of the processed grain foods. Once the outer shell is removed, the grain is tasty but has fewer nutrients than in its original form.

What would a registered dietitian say?

Aim to make about half of your daily choices whole grain and the other half from the refined grains group each day. This blend offers important nutrients from both whole and refined grains as well as more variety of taste and texture.

Quinoa, oats, wheat, and brown rice are common whole grains. Eaten in unprocessed forms, they are high in nutrients from the bran and germ. Refining and processing remove fiber, B vitamins, and other plant nutrients. Iron is also removed in processing, and that is how the necessity for fortification and enrichment of grains originated. *Fortified* and *enriched* are two terms you see on packages of processed grains. A good example of this labeling is all-purpose flour, which is enriched with iron, thiamine, folic acid, riboflavin, and niacin. Enriching flour came about in the 1940s when the US government decided that flour would be fortified to address beriberi and pellagra, both diseases caused by deficiencies of these nutrients. Later, folic acid was added to refined wheat flour to eliminate neural tube defects in the unborn.

Examples of Whole Grain Form of Food	Examples of Refined Grain Form of Food
Polenta made from coarse ground corn meal, 1/2 cup cooked	Corn meal instant grits, 1/2 cup cooked
Whole wheat bread, 1 slice	White bread, 1 slice
Whole wheat durum spaghetti, 1/2 cup cooked	Spaghetti, 1/2 cup cooked
Steel cut or whole oats, 1/2 cup cooked	1 packet of flavored oatmeal, cooked
Brown rice, 1/2 cup cooked	Converted white rice, 1/2 cup cooked
Whole wheat tortilla	White tortilla

Balance Between Whole Grains and Refined Grains

It comes as no surprise that our taste buds prefer refined, highly processed grains with a sweet taste and soft bite. Who does not like the mouthfeel of a sweet dinner roll? Americans get plenty of grains, but the grains we eat are mostly refined and come largely from white flour and rice, processed corn meals, and oats. But optimal cell health to fight off diseases like breast cancer or heart disease requires plant nutrients found in unrefined, unprocessed grains. Plant nutrients like selenium, which tamps down bad compounds in the cells, and phenolic acid, which boosts antioxidant power for heart health, are found in whole grains, like brown rice, but not in the white, refined forms.

Eating too much of the tasty, sweeter, softer versions of grains, especially white flour, and rice, has extended the tarnished reputation grains have had, along with many waistlines. The DGA states that at least half of the total grains eaten should be whole grains, with a daily goal of forty-eight grams. The other half should be enriched or fortified grains. According to these guidelines, up to half of the grains you eat should be refined to ensure that you get enough B vitamins, including folic acid and iron, nutrients that many do not get enough of from other foods. Refined grains are fortified and enriched with these hard-to-get nutrients, so an eating pattern without any refined grains falls short of these nutrients.

Caution is in order when applying the DGA's, due to the overabundance of refined grains on dinner plates and far fewer whole grains. Survivors will thrive with a smaller percentage of refined grains, such as 25 percent allowing for the enjoyment of a soft dinner roll or a thick slice of Texas toast, while the remaining 75 percent of breads and cereals are whole grain.

Making Sense of Grains: Definitions

- Fiber: A whole grain food is not necessarily high in fiber. A high-fiber food has five or more grams of fiber per serving. Fiber gives the grain structure and shape.

- A refined-grain food label will list enriched bleached flour or enriched long grain rice as the first ingredient. Refined grains are usually enriched with thiamine, riboflavin, niacin, or folic acid.

- A whole-grain food can be identified by the ingredient list on the food label. The whole grain should be the first ingredient—or the second ingredient. Whole grain foods usually have fewer ingredients overall.

- Fortified means that a nutrient your body needs is added to a food that may not have had this nutrient in the first place.

- Enriched means that original nutrients are added back into processed or refined foods.

Finding whole grain foods has become easier with the whole grain stamp (www.wholegrainscouncil.org). The labels, which are brown, black, and gold, indicate the percentage of whole grain content in crackers, breads, and cereals. Specifically, if a product bears the 100 percent whole grain stamp, then *all* its grain ingredients are *whole* grain, while one with a 50 percent stamp indicates that half of the grains are whole grains. Foods labeled with Basic means that less than 50 percent of the grains in the food are whole grains.

Confused? It's not easy to make sense of what makes a grain whole, refined, enriched, or fortified. And what about fiber? Isn't fiber important? Why would I choose a refined grain over one with fiber? What makes a high-fiber food? A few definitions for clarification are included in the graphic.

Take note of the refined grains description: fiber is not added back when grains are fortified. Fiber, as discussed previously, is good for decreasing inflammation, reducing the risk of several cancers, including breast and colon, maintaining heart health, and stabilizing blood sugar levels. Not all whole grains are high in fiber. Read the bread label carefully to note that a *high-fiber food* has three or more grams of fiber per serving. As an example to support label reading, a bread labeled "twelve-grain" would seemingly contain a lot of fiber. But a twelve-grain slice has one gram of fiber compared to whole wheat bread, which has four grams of fiber per slice. However, the twelve-grain bread is high in whole grains. The grains used in making bread determine the amount of fiber, not the whole grain label. As this applies to you and me, women fifty years and older need seventeen to twenty-eight grams of *fiber* daily, depending on calorie needs. Keep in mind that fiber comes from grains, vegetables, *and* fruits.

Finally, as a reminder, at least 50 percent of all the grains you eat should be whole grain, and the other half refined.

Eating more fiber will make you fuller for longer. This means you are less prone to visit a vending machine for a midafternoon snack or rifle through the cupboard just before the evening meal. To test this, eat whole wheat bread for a week and pay attention to how satisfied your belly feels. When we eat carbohydrates, which all grains are, and those carbohydrates are refined, our brains believe we need more. White flour

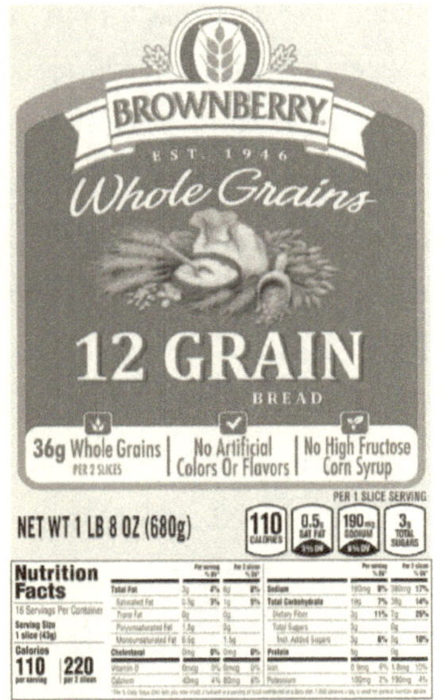

says, "I want more," and whole wheat flour says, "I am satisfied." Eating too many sweet, starchy foods sets in motion a carbohydrate craving followed by more carbohydrate snacking, leading to weight gain.[43] Experiment by trading out buttery crackers for a whole grain version or substitute yummy potato bread for a whole wheat version. You will notice you eat fewer whole grain varieties than refined versions.

Most Adults Do Not Get Enough Dairy Foods

As a teen, I worked at a local dairy, milking cows, cleaning pens, and feeding the calves. It is messy, stinky work, but I loved it. After work, the morning milking crew would gather 'round to sample the cream of the day. There is nothing like fresh cream straight from the cow. I am unapologetically biased in favor of milk, but I am smart enough to understand why others are not.

Since my days as a teenage milkmaid, dairy foods have been in the news for good and bad reasons. Dairy foods have been blamed for contributing to heart disease, high cholesterol, obesity, and environmental concerns. Foods go in and out of favor as studies reach journalists' desks, and a recent news headline stated that dairy milk, even in moderate amounts, increases the risk of breast cancer. Though a headline like this is unsettling, the American Institute for Cancer Research (AICR) responded with a message to regard this news trail with caution. After further analysis, cancer organizations concluded that when combined with other milk studies, there is no substantial evidence to suggest that dairy foods increase breast cancer risks. Other studies have raised concern about dairy foods, such as how drinking milk from cows treated with hormones can increase the risk of breast cancer. These studies failed to find a clear link, and currently, drinking milk produced with or without hormone treatments (which are used to increase milk production) is considered safe for women.[44]

Over the past two decades, people have eaten fewer dairy foods for various reasons, such as vegan diets and environmental concerns. Another likely cause for the decrease is that guidance has long suggested an avoidance of full-fat milk, cheese, and yogurt to decrease higher saturated fat. A study with over thirty thousand postmenopausal women set out to test whether this guidance bears truth by studying if dairy foods do indeed increase fats, lipids, insulin-related factors, and inflammatory markers that signal the onset of heart disease and diabetes. What they found contradicts older guidance to avoid or limit full-fat dairy foods. While the study cannot fully determine that dairy foods prevent disease, this information points to research that further substantiates the nutritional value of dairy foods. In fact, the results suggest that except for butter, a higher intake of dairy foods is connected to more favorable lab values for blood sugar, lipids (cholesterol), and inflammation markers.[45]

Butter did not fare well; eating too much of it tends to increase cholesterol levels due to butter's concentrated saturated fat content. On the other hand, low-fat yogurt increases the healthy (HDL) type of cholesterol. To save calories, consuming lower-fat dairy foods (and limiting butter!) is a prudent approach, but this study suggests there is a neutral effect on heart disease and diabetes risk from both lower- and full-fat dairy foods. Experts who seek to find mechanisms for how food impacts disease hypothesize that fermented dairy, such as yogurt and cheese, may favorably alter gut microbiome diversity and, as such, offer a possible link in how dairy foods may prevent heart disease and diabetes.

Some women prefer to buy organic dairy foods for higher levels of certain nutrients, notably conjugated linoleic acid, a cancer-fighting antioxidant believed to help decrease body fat. Organically produced dairy foods are also popular for the elimination of antibiotics and hormones. Keep in mind that all dairy foods are fortified with vitamin D, which is necessary for calcium absorption.

The bottom line is that dairy may have a protective role in preventing heart disease and diabetes through a pathway that regulates insulin response and, therefore, inflammation, which you learned a bit about in "Food as Medicine." Overall, this new evidence removes some of the bad reputation that dairy foods have had in recent decades.

Research presented in the DGA suggests that 90 percent of US adults do not meet the recommended three servings of dairy per day, and only 20 percent of adults drink milk as a beverage daily.[46] Commonly consumed dairy foods like ice cream, frozen yogurt, flavored milk, cheese with pasta, pizza, sandwich slices, and sweetened yogurt are high in saturated fat, sodium, or added sugars. Although this list of foods does contain dairy, dietitians like me tend to think that the good stuff, like calcium and vitamin D that your bones need, phosphorus for energy production, and a high-value protein that keeps your muscles strong, is canceled out by sodium, added sugars, and higher overall fat. These nutrients are found abundantly in low-fat or skim milk, plain yogurt, and lower-fat cheese without excessive saturated fats. To recap, choose some dairy foods like full-fat milk, and choose others with lower fat, such as low-fat yogurt, to balance out the calories. Few foods offer the variety of benefits found in dairy; for you and your bone health, the amount of calcium in three servings per day is hard to get from non-dairy foods. (Chapter 6, "In the Pink," will address bone health in greater detail.)

Alternative Milks—Better Than Dairy?

As a dietitian, I appreciate how nutrition facts tell an undeniable truth. Dairy foods are better in several ways than the alternative milks, at least by nutrient standards. An important nutrition detail to consider is protein.

The protein found in dairy foods is more digestible and available for breakdown and has a superior amino acid makeup in comparison to the forms of protein found in alternative milk beverages. The other important factor is calcium, which you need to prevent bone thinning caused by aromatase inhibitors and aging in general. Vitamin D, as mentioned, is needed for absorption of both calcium and phosphorus. Dairy milk naturally contains calcium and is fortified with vitamin D. Alternative milks are fortified with both calcium and vitamin D.

People choose alternative milk for many reasons, including a plant-based eating plan such as vegan or vegetarian, food allergies, lactose intolerance, saturated fat content, hormones and antibiotics, low carbon footprint concerns, and animal welfare. These milks are made from soy, almond, potato, cashew, flax, hemp, oats, peas, coconut, and rice. Each of these milk alternative products is processed differently. For example, these milks may have rice syrup, barley malt, or cane sugar as sweeteners, as well as water, food additives, and thickeners, like carrageenan (seaweed) or sunflower lecithin to give these beverages a taste and mouthfeel like dairy milk. According to the USDA database, nut milks are diluted with water, and many have added sugars depending on whether they are unsweetened or sweetened. Milk alternatives, except soy milk, have less protein and are enriched with calcium.

Comparison of Dairy and Milk Alternatives

Milk	Dairy	Almond	Soy	Oat	Rice
Calories	100	40	100	120	120
Grams, Protein	8	1	7-8	1-4	1
Milligrams, calcium	300	432*	300*	460*	300*
% RDA of calcium	25	36	25	38	25
Grams, sugar added	0	11	0-8	7-19	10
Water added	no	yes	yes	yes	yes

1200mg calcium = recommended daily allowance (RDA).
**Enriched with calcium. 4 grams of added sugar = 1 teaspoon of sugar.*
Information compiled from USDA Foods Database.
www.fns.usda.gov/usda-foods-database.

Among the alternative milks, only soy qualifies as a suitable substitute meeting the DGA recommendation for dairy because soy has a similar nutrient profile as dairy for a high-quality, easily digested protein not found in the others. The other alternative milks do not meet the dairy group recommendations due to added sugars and lower protein content. For those with milk allergies or lactose intolerance, a milk alternative, other than dairy or soy, is a suitable, although less desirable, option because of lower protein content. Lactose-free milk contains a similar calcium profile to that of regular dairy milk for those with lactose intolerance. Soy, the least processed of alternative milks, is fortified with calcium, plus vitamins A and D. And soy milk is a whole soy food and considered safe for breast cancer survivors. If it is important to you, bear in mind that soybeans have the most genetically modified organisms (GMOs) among these alternatives, but this can be easily addressed by purchasing a certified non-GMO brand.

Mix and Match Protein

Much has been written about meat, with some reports proclaiming meat as ideal for protein while other articles paint a picture of meat as bad for health. The truth is somewhere in between. Healing of the body after injury, surgery, and cancer treatments requires adequate protein, which does not need to come from animal protein alone. Organs and muscles need a steady supply of protein to maintain function and repair themselves. Protein from the foods we eat provides the building blocks for all structures in our body. But Americans consume more than the recommended amounts of animal protein. Mixing and matching animal and plant proteins is a good compromise for better health.

The DGA suggests that adults get five ounces of protein daily, preferably a combination of red meat, poultry, eggs, and seafood, and a blend of nuts, seeds, and soy. Dairy foods, as you learned previously, contain protein too. Consider the benefits of eating a mixture of protein sources to make up the recommended five ounces:

- A shift toward eating more protein foods from seafood, beans, peas, and lentils provides protein and offers healthy omega-3 fatty acids from fish, especially salmon, and fiber from beans.
- Replacing processed or high-fat meats (e.g., hot dogs, sausages, bacon) with seafood or beans helps lower fat and salt intake.

As with other food groups, most of us have room for improvement. Seventy-five percent of Americans eat more than the recommended servings of meat, poultry, and eggs. About 90 percent of the protein Americans eat comes from casseroles, pizza, pasta dishes, and sandwiches—which, as you are beginning to understand, are high in processed starches, saturated fat, salt, and calories. Recent studies linking a high intake of red meat—such as beef, lamb, pork, and processed meat—with colon cancer have resulted in a recommendation to limit red meat intake to twelve to eighteen ounces (cooked) per week and to avoid consuming any processed meats, which includes ham, bacon, and hot dogs.[47] Current recommendations do not limit chicken, turkey, fish, or low-fat dairy foods.

Animal protein from beef, pork, lamb, and chicken has high biological value for the human body. Our digestive system is well-suited to breaking down and absorbing protein and iron from animal sources. And animal protein contains the right blend of amino acids that our body needs. Iron from animal meats is the most absorbable form of iron available for the human digestive system. In contrast to what you just read about approval for a limited amount of saturated fat found in dairy foods, animal meats, notably beef, lamb, and pork, do not get the same approval, however. Eating too much red meat means consuming far too much saturated fat, and as such, the best advice is to limit red meat to several times per week, not every day.

Ninety percent of Americans do not meet the DGA's recommended amounts of seafood. Fish is high in protein and lower in fat, and some offer omega-3 fatty acids, which our bodies cannot produce. The cost of fish is often an issue for food budgets, but eating canned or frozen tuna and salmon once or twice weekly is an affordable option. Finally, more than half of us fall short of the recommended amounts of seeds, nuts, and soy foods. Eating more beans, at least once weekly, diminishes the amount of saturated fat (and calories!) while also saving money. Sprinkling nuts and seeds on a salad is another way to add protein and move toward more meatless meals. A mix-and-match approach to protein sources is a fitting tactic to incorporate more meatless, vegetarian-style meals using fish, lentils, beans, or tofu for a wider variety of nutrients, lower fat intake, better heart health, and improved weight management.

A Beef about Beef

A few words to get in on the beef about beef. All beef, grass-fed or conventionally grown with grains, is high in iron, zinc, B vitamins, and of course, protein. Concerns about soil erosion and richness, water quality, animal welfare, and antibiotic use have made grass-fed beef a popular option, but aside from saturated fat content, the overall nutrition of both grass-fed and grain-fed beef offers high-quality protein plus iron.

Meat in general is a good source of B12, or cobalamin, needed for the normal metabolism of cells. Survivors older than sixty-five years are at risk for a B12 deficiency due to digestive changes with aging, and they may need a supplement. A variety of healthy protein choices are available to suit your personal taste preferences and your budget.

Cancer organizations have, in recent years, continued to lower the number of recommended amounts for red meat (beef, pork, and lamb). For example, AICR suggests eating twelve to eighteen ounces *per week* of red meat, and the American Cancer Society (ACS) recommends generally limiting red meat. For a woman who needs 1,500 calories per day and requires five ounces of meat protein per day, she could, for example, eat a combination of meats including beef, chicken, and eggs. A medium-size hamburger is three ounces, and an egg is another one to two ounces (depending on whether it's a small or jumbo size), which fulfills her meat protein needs for a day.

To limit saturated fat in steaks or burgers, choose grass-fed beef. Grass-fed beef is not guaranteed organic, but it lacks the hormones and antibiotics used in conventional grain-fed beef and has less cholesterol-raising fats, slightly more omega-3 fatty acids, and less saturated fat than grain-fed.

The beef about beef will continue, but for survivors, eating red meat a few times a week is acceptable. All the hullabaloo comes from research showing that *daily* red meat can do more harm than good while also arising from concerns about the millions of Americans who, despite recommendations, continue to eat beef every day and sometimes at each meal. As a smart survivor making good choices about meat protein, aim to eat beef one to two times per week and then choose chicken and eggs to meet weekly meat protein needs.

What would a registered dietitian say?

Meat burned or smoked during preparation has high amounts of cancer-causing compounds (heterocyclic amines and polycyclic aromatic hydrocarbons). Limit or avoid these. Marinating meats before cooking and cooking at a lower temperature avoids these compounds.

What Is All the Cluck about Chicken?

The marketing for chicken is befuddling. Lower in fat than beef or pork (if not fried), high in iron if you choose the dark meat, and packed with protein, chicken is a wise addition to your eating pattern. The confusion begins with questions about organic, free range, and conventionally grown chicken.

To shed some light on the hen house, know that all chickens raised and produced for meat in the US are cage-free and hormone-free but not necessarily free range. Large, commercial poultry production facilities are known to use antibiotics as a preventive measure against disease, whereas a smaller producer may not administer antibiotics to the flock. Presently, to address antibiotic resistance concerns, large producers are incorporating different methods for maintaining the health of the peep without antibiotics. In any case, the nutrient profile for chicken is the same regardless of how they are raised. Food budget, food beliefs, and preferences will guide your purchasing choice of chicken.

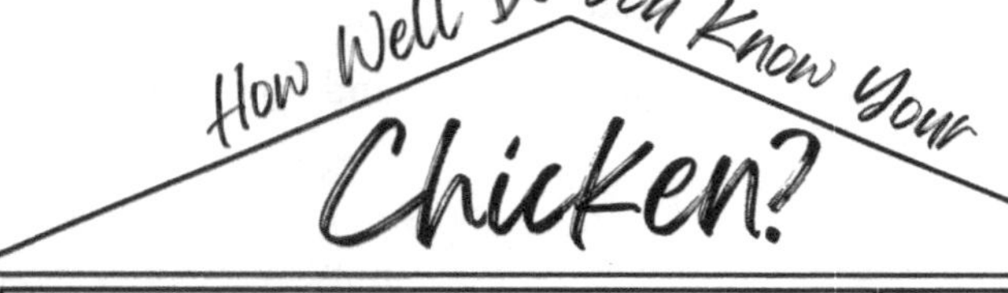

VEGETARIAN Chickens are fed a meatless diet. A vegetarian diet requires savvy nutrient balancing and culinary satisfaction for chickens on the part of chicken producers. Chickens are omnivores and they prefer both meat and plant foods.

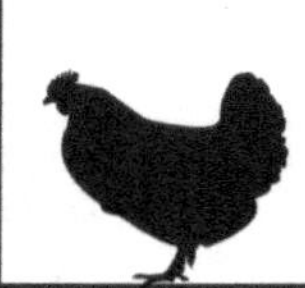

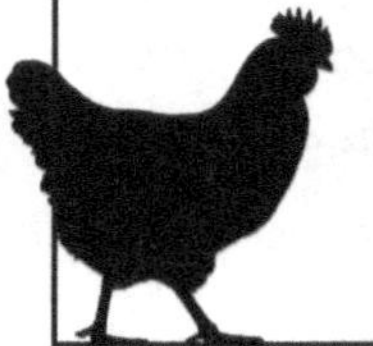

ORGANIC Chickens receive one dose of antibiotics on their first day of life to prevent disease. Organic chicken contains no other antibiotics or pesticides. USDA Organic means chicken is fed a vegetarian, non-GMO diet. Certification requirements increase the price.

ANTIBIOTIC-FREE Chickens means antibiotics given are for disease prevention and enhanced feed efficiency only at birth. Prior to slaughter, the bird undergoes a withdrawal period without any antibiotics.

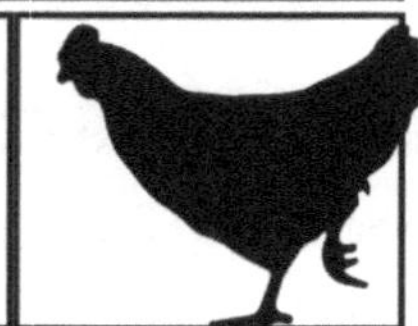

Cracking Open the Truth about Eggs

Since the 1960s, the truth about eggs has been scrambled by concerns about cholesterol and heart health, but since 2015, nutrition experts agree there is no available evidence showing a strong connection between foods, including eggs, containing cholesterol and your cholesterol levels. The DGA includes eggs among the list of nutrient-dense protein foods, and the American Heart Association no longer recommends limiting cholesterol to 300 milligrams or less per day. Eggs go over easy in health benefits for survivors, including:

- **Overall health**: Get cracking and eat the yolk! Nearly half of an egg's protein and most of the vitamins and minerals, including those supporting the body and brain, are in the yolk.
- **Bone health**: Eggs are the only food naturally containing vitamin D, which works with calcium for bone maintenance.
- **Boost brain power**: As one of the best sources of choline, eggs support lifelong brain health at every age and stage by bolstering memory, thinking, and moods.
- **Muscle and weight**: With six to eight grams of protein per egg, muscle health is optimized and you feel satisfied without overeating.

Younger, healthier survivors can eat up to one egg per day, while older Americans can eat up to two eggs per day. As an inexpensive and convenient source of protein with numerous vitamins and minerals, eggs are an economical, nutrient-dense choice, particularly with a tight budget.

Take a Pass on Salt

A section focusing on salt may feel as out of place here as it would if you discovered a highly skilled French chef frying hamburgers on the grill at a backyard barbecue. Recall, however, that making every bite count implies choosing foods that are nutrient-dense and shunning foods that are high in salt. This approach tracks well with making every bite count. Furthermore, with an eye on avoiding heart disease and high blood pressure aggravated by high-sodium foods, breast cancer survivors benefit from taking a pass on the saltshaker.

What would a registered dietitian say?

Drink eight tall glasses of water each day and reduce salt intake to avoid weight gain. A study by Richard Johnson, a professor of medicine at the University of Colorado, found that dehydration plus a high salt intake alters how food is broken down, which results in more fat storage, contributing to a person becoming overweight or obese.[48]

Like ketchup and mustard go with burgers and hot dogs, saturated fat and salt (sodium) go with a risk of heart disease. High sodium, or salt, intake is linked to high blood pressure. Just like guidelines for saturated fats, the American Heart Association has something to say about sodium as it relates to heart health and high blood pressure. A decrease in salt intake decreases blood pressure and reduces heart disease.[49] As recommended by the American Heart Association, Americans should aim to consume no more than 2,300 milligrams (mg) of sodium a day. An ideal limit is no more than 1,500 mg per day for most adults, particularly those with high blood pressure. Americans eat a lot of salt, over three thousand mg on average, so cutting back by a thousand mg a day improves blood pressure and heart health.

How Much Salt Are You Eating?

With a mere teaspoon containing 2,300 milligrams of sodium, salt intake adds up quickly. Sodium chloride, or table salt, is approximately 40 percent sodium. It's important to understand just how much sodium is in salt so you can take measures to control your intake.

- 1/4 teaspoon salt = 575 mg sodium
- 1/2 teaspoon salt = 1,150 mg sodium
- 3/4 teaspoon salt = 1,725 mg sodium
- 1 teaspoon salt = 2,300 mg sodium

The saltshaker is not your biggest problem. A food with more than five hundred milligrams of sodium is a high-sodium food, and yet many foods have 250 milligrams or more, and since these are frequently consumed, the average daily salt intake is 3,400 milligrams,[50] roughly one and a half times more than the 2,300 milligrams currently recommended and more than two times the ideal of 1,500 milligrams. Processed and convenience foods, as well as those eaten while dining out, are the big culprits. Restaurants are known for the generous use of saltshakers, and as such, cooking at home more often is the best way to consume less sodium. So, take a pass on salt and eat at home as often as possible. Take it a step further and regularly read the Nutrition Facts label to help you choose foods with less sodium, reduced sodium, or no salt added, and flavor foods with herbs and spices instead of salt. You will find that some food brands are lower in sodium than others.

Laurie's Top 12 High Salt Foods

1. Cold cuts, hot dogs, sausage, ham, jerky, and bacon

2. Tomato juices and sauces, unless labeled otherwise

3. Salted snacks: pretzels, chips (potato, tortilla), salted nuts, crackers

4. Bottled salad dressings, BBQ sauce, cocktail sauce

5. Packaged mixes for noodle, potato, and rice side dishes

6. Processed cheese and cheese spreads

7. Frozen entrees and pot pies

8. Canned soup

9. Pickles

10. Instant pudding mix

11. Cottage cheese

12. Pizza

A Grain of Wisdom: Iodized Salt and Breast Cancer

A salt or sodium deficiency is rare in America due to the use of salt for flavoring in processed foods, but like other minerals, correct amounts are critical for body functions. Sodium is necessary for nerve and muscle function, normal cell operations, and the acid-base balance of blood; therefore, consuming the right type and quantity of salt is important. Following the popular food trend of using sea salt in your cooking could mean you are missing out on iodine, a mineral associated with thyroid function. Sea salt is favored by chefs for a crunchy, coarse texture and stronger flavor when added to foods, and some people prefer sea salt because it is natural, but sea and table salts are both naturally derived. Believed to also be lower in sodium because of its larger crystals, this common notion about a lower-sodium content when using sea salt is inaccurate. Although sea salt has larger crystal sizes, meaning there are fewer crystals in a measuring spoon, both sea salt and iodized table salt have about the same amount of sodium per teaspoon or about 2,300 milligrams.

Created by the evaporation of sea water, sea salt naturally contains calcium, magnesium, and potassium, as well as a small amount of iodine, but it does not offer a superior health benefit over iodized table salt. Iodized table salt is mined from salt quarries, and during processing, iodine is added, and then the salt is ground into fine crystals for maximum absorption in foods and drinks. But, eating too little iodized salt may have an impact on breast health, especially in younger women.[51] Iodine is important for the development of healthy breast tissue. Notably, inadequate iodine in the diet is associated with fibrocystic breast disease (dense breasts), which affects about half of the women of childbearing age. Fibrous, dense breasts are linked to an increased risk of developing breast cancer.

Iodine plays a role in an organ we do not often think about—our thyroid. The thyroid is a small, butterfly-shaped gland found at the base of your neck, just below your Adam's apple. This gland makes the thyroid hormone that travels in your blood to all parts of your body. The thyroid hormone controls the breakdown and absorption of food, including how fast you burn calories and the beating of your heart. Importantly, women are more likely than men to have thyroid diseases, especially after pregnancy and menopause, and a healthy thyroid requires iodine intake. This is another reason to make sure you and your female family members are getting enough iodized salt. Sea salt is okay for occasional use, but regular use of iodized salt is important for breast and overall health. Food sources of iodine include:

- iodine-rich seaweed
- dairy
- fish
- eggs
- iodine-enriched grain products
- plant foods grown in iodine-rich soil

More Pieces of the Survivor Puzzle: Kathy

Kathy was diagnosed with breast cancer in her right breast, requiring surgery, chemotherapy, and radiation; her treatment course and transition to active survivorship were challenging. Kathy's recovery from treatment was complicated by a history of depression and weight gain.

During treatments, others would remark on her bravery, but she did not feel brave. Barely getting by, she kept her diagnosis at an arm's distance so she could fight. After active treatments were complete, Kathy joined a weight loss group for other breast cancer survivors. Within the group, she found encouragement, and the group pulled her along, validating her efforts to improve her weight and stick to her plans for more walking. She lost a modest amount of weight, began to feel better, and despite achy knees, she started walking more. Her depressive symptoms improved.

The support group was interrupted by the COVID-19 pandemic. Kathy's support network was no longer at arm's reach, and she regained weight, falling back into her moods. Then two years later, a visit to a cardiologist revealed that she had heart issues requiring surgery and ongoing treatments. With a strong family history of heart disease, she was aware of the consequences but was caught off guard at the news of her heart problems.

After the surgery, Kathy became discouraged and resistant to further advice to take charge of her health and amend her lifestyle habits. Deep down, Kathy felt punished by her breast cancer, heart disease, and painful knees, all of which she felt were a result of being overweight. Then, during a visit to the beach to be with her sister, she had chest pains requiring a trip to the Emergency Department. That scare got her attention and snapped her out of resistance to self-care.

When she returned home, she put sticky notes all over her house with statistics about women and heart disease. These reminders loosened the denial she felt about her health conditions. Then, her six-year-old granddaughter asked her with "loving honesty" if she had lost some weight so that she could be healthier. Ashamed but now more motivated, Kathy found both her social-driven purpose—her granddaughter—as well as a health-driven purpose to address heart problems. With greater resolve from her purposes, she broke out of her slump, settling into working toward weight loss, better eating habits, and more physical movement. With greater determination, she started over with diet and physical activity. Now more aware of the need to cut out sodium and lose weight, she considered rejoining a weight loss group to help better track food intake and approach eating with more purpose and direction. After starting and failing repeatedly, Kathy realized that it takes a lot longer to find and feel success, particularly after cancer and heart disease. Now she sees her repeated failed attempts at weight loss and better eating habits as another reason to get it right. This time around, she set her sights on a smaller, more manageable weight loss goal that comes with an emphasis on heart-healthy foods and more attention to portion sizes rather than a rigid recording of every food. All of this is her path toward dancing happily around her kitchen more often and with a lighter step.

Working with Kathy and many others like her has been my life's greatest accomplishment. Experience and studies have shown me that not one survivor is like any other in terms of their health history and individual nutrient needs. My own diagnosis clarified for me that each survivor desires a lighter, more personal touch to nutritional guidance. There is no one-size-fits-all approach that works, nor is there a timeline that a survivor must adhere to for success.

Kathy resisted self-care for months but gradually made her way forward with the sticky notes and a recognition that small changes lead to getting it right.

Here, I demonstrate what Kathy's nutritional care plan looks like. In this plan, look for signs of food as medicine, puzzle pieces, a soft-as-a-feather approach to changes, and progress, not perfection. Of note, the focus was on Kathy's heart health challenges, which led to discussions about her vegetarian eating style and how to adjust it for more anti-inflammatory power by eating more vegetables and fruits and switching to whole grain pasta. Eating out, as well as using frozen convenience foods, increased Kathy's daily sodium intake. A review with a handout from the American Heart Association on ways to reduce sodium reminded her to eat at home more often and read labels for sodium content. As for physical activity, her cardiologist arranged for her attendance at cardiac rehabilitation.

Laurie's Nutritional Consult with Kathy

BIO	KATHY: 65 years old, married, grown kids, grandkids		
Kathy Desires	Weight loss, improved eating choices for managing heart disease		
Health History	Breast cancer, heart disease, depression, overweight/obese		
Weight	195 pounds	Height	5'5"
Body Mass Index	32.4	Waist Circumference	38
Food Allergies	None	Physical Activity	Light to moderate
Food Prep Skills	Prefers simple recipes		
Current Eating Pattern	Vegetarian, high in salt with pre-packaged foods, favors lots of pasta.		
KATHY'S NUTRITIONAL CARE PLAN			
Daily calorie range for weight loss:	1,450 – 1,550	Recommended Eating Pattern	Heart-healthy vegetarian-Mediterranean
Goals	1. Lower-sodium food choices, goal of 1,500–2,300 milligrams/day 2. Vegetarian, heart-healthy food choices		
Materials Provided to Support	• Sodium Content in Foods • How to Reduce Sodium. • Vegetarian-Mediterranean food pyramid and resources reviewed.		

DIETITIAN NOTES

Kathy and I looked at American Heart Association eating patterns. Kathy chose to continue using a Mediterranean-Vegetarian style for the heart healthy foods she wants and needs. Reviewed how to reduce salt in her food choices and food preparation. I reminded her that these changes will not come quickly, and she should allow 2–3 months to get "good at this" and discussed how gradual weight loss will come with more emphasis on lower-calorie foods, more fruits/vegetables, less pasta. Scheduled a follow-up visit for one month. For now, there is a priority for choosing lower-sodium foods and using the Vegetarian-Mediterranean eating plan to begin to guide her meal and snack choices.

Next visit: See how she's doing with lower-sodium foods, vegetarian eating plans, and recommended B12 and iron. Will talk about tracking calories, slow gradual weight loss, and finding a supportive weight-management group.

Fitting All the Puzzle Pieces Together

You are now more ready to assemble pieces of your puzzle. At this point, you may wonder which eating pattern matches up to your plans for a healthier eating style. In "Food as Medicine," you learned that breast cancer survivors are at risk for cancer recurrence and also heart disease and diabetes. Further, you learned how anti-inflammatory eating patterns work to prevent chronic inflammation, which is connected to the formation of these diseases. A sizable piece of the puzzle you are completing is more familiarity with eating styles that emphasize overall health.

Twenty years ago, nutrition experts believed that diabetes, heart disease, and others required specific diets to prevent or control these illnesses. Today, though, more evidence points toward a common thread, with individual tweaks for some, to avoid and manage these diseases. Shared guidance includes limiting or avoiding alcohol, adding more emphasis on fruits and vegetables, and decreasing junk foods. There are numerous plant-based eating pattern options like Dietary Approaches to Stop Hypertension (the DASH eating style), Diabetes Risk Reduction (DRRD) (mentioned earlier in this chapter), the Mediterranean, My Plate, low-carbohydrate, vegetarian, and others that are balanced with all four food groups. Again, there are slight modifications for various disease conditions, but what these eating styles share is a plant-based foundation.

You could choose any of the eating patterns listed and take comfort in the sensibility of your anti-inflammatory approach. The good news is that the same lifestyle activities that help us avoid another bout of breast cancer also help keep us free from heart disease and diabetes. Fittingly, the seven priority food categories chosen for the In the Pink Plate Plan featured in chapter 7—dark green vegetables, red and orange vegetables, beans/peas/lentils, fruits, dairy, seafood, and nuts/seeds/soy—mirror the plant-based, anti-inflammatory eating styles while emphasizing the nutritional needs of breast cancer survivors.

You will learn more about choosing and balancing monounsaturated, polyunsaturated, and saturated fats in chapter 6. This chapter also looks at follow-up visits with Kathy and highlights how a sound nutritional care plan is designed, progressively helping her to place together puzzle pieces that work for her health issues and food preferences. A happier dance through life, no matter how old you are or how challenging your health issues are, is what you want. It would give me great satisfaction if I could wave a wand and make you healthier, but this is impossible. You must do the work to get to a place where your steps are lighter, the music faster, and the joy much greater. Only you can decide how the pieces of your puzzle fit together. By placing one small piece together with another, and then another, you complete your own healthier life masterpiece.

Physical activity is yet another piece of the puzzle. The next chapter, "Glisten," explores ways to add physical activity safely and comfortably to your daily life.

KEY POINTS

- Both weight and eating patterns determine your risk for cancer recurrence, heart disease, and diabetes.

- All four food groups contain unique nutrients necessary for overall health. Fruits and vegetables offer plant nutrients. A sensible balance of whole and refined grains both nourishes and satisfies. Dairy foods support bone health. A mix-and-match approach to protein sources is a fitting way to eat well.

- Cancer, heart disease, and diabetes are connected to inflammation, and all three of these diseases can be prevented or managed with lifestyle changes such as weight loss and anti-inflammatory eating patterns.

Glisten

"Good things come to those
who GLISTEN."

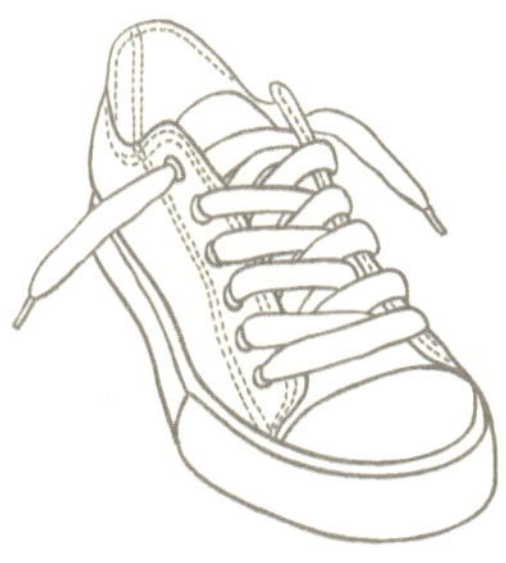

BEFORE MY WORK AS A CANCER DIETITIAN, I was an exercise instructor working in a variety of fitness facilities, including cardiac rehabilitation, a YMCA, a university physical fitness department, and a women's health center. My niche was to lead women, mostly ages forty and over, toward greater fitness through aerobic dance, resistance training, and inspiration. Among this group, most participants had conversations alluding to the fact that they dreaded the sweat, but one, Mimi, referred to her perspiration as "glistening." Hers was a shimmering representation of a joyful embrace of physical movement. Meanwhile, others expressed disdain and drudgery, keeping a watchful eye on the clock for the end of the class. For most participants, creativity, good music, and sensitivity to their abilities were far more important than any dance moves I had planned. What these women wanted most was to just "get it done" and sweat, but not too much, then get on with their day. My classes ended with each participant making a mental checkmark on their day: Exercise, check.

I have seen and heard many descriptions of how women feel about exercise. Some women delight in a sopping sweat as they bop in a dance exercise class, while others are disgusted with sweat trickling down their faces while they walk the neighborhood. Some women grimace with pain when they move more. We are all different in how we feel about physical movement. Exercise makes me feel empowered, capable, and gritty, especially now that I am a survivor. Sweating gives me a can-do spirit and reminds me that I am doing my best to take care of myself. The struggles I have with surgical changes that resulted in left arm and shoulder pain are not leaving anytime soon. More stretching makes this more tolerable, but there are still things I can no longer do without pain. Through trial and error, I have found what works for me. The side effects that you have from treatment may make the thought of physical activity scary. Trying to make an exercise plan on your own may lead to painful aftereffects a day or two later. A key to moving more is first understanding how much movement you need and then figuring out which exercise plan fits with your ability and any lingering side effects.

Exercise may be a dirty word for you. I use the terms *physical movement* or *activity* as a way of removing the undesirable term "exercise." Physical activity involves walking to the store or mowing the lawn and is aptly defined as body movements that require increased energy expenditure. *Exercise* is defined as body movements that require increased energy expenditure and are planned, structured, and repeated with the goal of improving fitness. My guess is that it is the planned, structured, and repeated part that makes exercise undesirable. Physical activity is a part of everyday things we do. It may be that doing more of our everyday things is enough.

Breast Cancer Survivors Are a Booming Group

Breast cancer survivors are growing in number due to better screening and treatment methods. Popularly called "surthrivers" on social media groups, breast cancer survivors will potentially lead the way in understanding how more physical activity transforms how long and well you and I survive. By 2029, cancer survivors are expected to exceed twenty-one million people, and more than 60 percent of this group are and will continue to be over sixty-five years old.[52] The five-year survival rate for breast cancer exceeds 90 percent, while a 67 percent survival rate applies to all cancers.[53] Accordingly, based on this high five-year survival rate, breast cancer survivors comprise a sizable portion of all cancer survivors.[54] However, many of us are well into our sixties and struggle with the usual aches and pains of aging in addition to the challenges of side effects, like tender knees, lymphedema, numb feet and hands, loss of muscle, and arm pain resulting from treatments. Making the best of our remaining years requires some strong, somewhat difficult to swallow, medicine.

Physical activity and exercise are potent medicines, particularly when performed regularly. According to the American Cancer Society (ACS), American College of Sports Medicine (ACSM), and American Institute for Cancer Research (AICR), limiting sedentary behavior, such as sitting, lying down, watching TV, or other screen-based entertainment, is one of the most impactful changes a cancer survivor can perform.[55] Studies show that less than 10 percent of cancer survivors are active during surgery, chemotherapy, and radiation, and this does not change much once we have completed treatment.[56] AICR estimates that 30 percent of breast cancer recurrences and deaths are preventable with lifestyle changes, one of which is improving eating styles, and the other is engaging in regular physical activity.[57] But you need not sign up to run a marathon to consider yourself physically active. Yoga, walking, dancing, cycling, swimming, tai chi, gardening, and weight-lifting are acceptable forms of activity. An active lifestyle means some form of moving for some period every day. My favorite knowledge nugget from numerous physical activity studies for survivors is that even if you did not exercise before diagnosis, you gain benefits by beginning after your diagnosis. It is never too late to get more active. While I am unable to provide you with an individual activity plan in this book, this chapter will:

- present you with a better understanding of the impact physical activity has on your overall health and risk of breast cancer recurrence;
- help you identify how you can safely and capably become more physically active; and
- help you gain an appreciation for activity "prescriptions" created by cancer exercise professionals, and give you an example of a weekly physical activity plan for a beginner.

Physical Activity Is a Polypill

Nearly a thousand physical activity and cancer studies led health professionals to believe that regular and consistent movement is like a "polypill" that reduces the risks of a long list of ailments and diseases: heart disease, high blood pressure and stroke, metabolic syndrome, type 2 diabetes, breast cancer, colon cancer, depression, and of course, falls.[58]

Trends among cancer survivors suggest that 35 percent of all female cancer survivors report no physical activity. This percentage goes up in women who are sixty-five years and older. The older we get, the less active we are and the more we sit. The ACS and ACSM organizations recommend moderate activity for thirty minutes per day on five days each week for cancer survivors who are physically able. In fact, these recommendations are for all Americans.

Despite emerging evidence and these professional guidelines, activity recommendations are not a standard topic with your oncologist. This stems from several factors, the most notable a lack of reimbursement for cancer activity programs, and the other a shortage of safe, effective programs that address the needs of older and weaker survivors with other illnesses besides cancer.[59] I strongly advocate for physical activity, and not just because I do not mind sweating. It is because I want you to appreciate the benefits of moving more and sitting less, regardless of age and abilities.

It is not a stretch to say that if your oncologist could bottle up pills containing the recommended amount of physical activity per week, she would certainly prescribe it for you. Current recommendations for survivors and all Americans are:

- Engage in 150 minutes of moderate exercise each week or seventy-five minutes of vigorous physical activity per week.
- In addition, do two days of resistance workouts (hand weights, resistance bands)

- For more benefit, increase moderate physical activity to three hundred minutes per week.

Physical activity is powerful. In 2013, a breast cancer lifestyle researcher determined that the lifestyle factor most strongly and consistently associated with both breast cancer incidence and breast cancer recurrence risk is physical activity. He and his team determined that moderate recreational physical activity (such as three to four hours of walking per week) may reduce breast cancer incidence and that women with early-stage breast cancer who increase or maintain their physical activity may have lower recurrence risk as well.[60] The value of increased physical activity and weight loss in women with early-stage breast cancer is established by this study and others. (More about how physical activity enhances the quality of life for higher-risk cancers later in the chapter.)

The One-Two Punch of Moving More and Eating Better

The long list of survivors whom I have counseled delivers an important observation: survivors prefer a sensible, lower-calorie eating pattern over more physical activity. Adopting a fitness plan requires stepping out of daily schedules. Recall in "Trade Old Habits for Better Ones" that you do not "have to" exercise, but you do have to eat, and as such, adopting a new physical activity routine is more challenging than altering mealtime regimens. Yet choosing to embrace an anti-inflammatory eating pattern without incorporating more physical activity, too, is a missed opportunity. Ultimately, skipping out on activity means you are missing the powerful one-two punch packed into moving more and eating better. The two are like a horse and carriage; one pulls while the other provides the push to keep going.

Recall an earlier discussion about how weight loss decreases one's recurrence risk; this occurs because a reduced weight results in lower estrogen levels. This is particularly true for estrogen-positive cancer. If you are postmenopausal, have been physically inactive, and followed a high-calorie diet for many years, combining better eating and more movement delivers the "punch" you need to improve health. A 2018 study found that while a calorie-reduced eating style leads to weight loss, loss of muscle mass often follows, leading to weakness, reduced heart and lung function, poor bone health, and other issues. In a similar fashion, physical activity alone does not reduce estrogen to the same level as the one-two punch of eating better with more physical movement. However, this study found that if a reduced-calorie eating pattern is combined with physical activity, you add muscle, improve heart function, and reduce estrogen levels.[61] What I like about sharing this information with you is that no matter how inactive you have been or how unfavorable your diet has been, your health will benefit from the mixture of a lower-calorie diet and more physical activity. This is especially true for those who are overweight and out of shape. For postmenopausal women of normal weight, the improvement is beneficial but less dramatic because lowering estrogen involves decreasing body fat where estrogen is stored.

What would a registered dietitian say?

Do you think of calories burned during exercise in the same way as making a cash withdrawal at the bank? Do you believe an immediate weight loss should appear on the scale after workouts? If only it were that simple. More precisely, physical activity maintains your weight, including any recent weight loss. With regular physical activity, you build muscle and increase calories burned for several hours after your workout is complete, keeping your weight steady.

Researchers over the past decade or so have shown an increased interest in how physical activity changes hormones in the body. Some hormones such as insulin, sex hormones like estrogen, and those that regulate appetite and food consumption are of interest because of the educated belief that if you can improve the levels of these hormones in your body, you lose the moderate 5–10 percent amount of weight that is shown to decrease the risk of diseases. Leptin, often featured as a weight-loss topic in the media, is one of these hormones. Lower levels of leptin result in lower appetite, less food intake, and weight loss. Another hormone, adiponectin, adjusts how well insulin works and has anti-inflammation properties. Researchers theorize that when combined, weight loss and exercise lead to more favorable levels of these hormones than if women just lose weight or only exercise or do neither.[62]

A large study consisting of four hundred overweight and obese women was divided into four groups of one hundred participants in an effort to examine how the combination of a weight loss eating pattern and physical activity leads to better levels of these hormones.[63] Each woman was assigned to one of four groups: physical activity alone, weight loss diet alone, diet plus physical activity, or no changes to diet or exercise. Researchers discovered that the women in the diet-plus-physical-activity group lost more than 10 percent of their original weight over one year. This was significantly more than the other three groups. Importantly, this combination group also had the greatest decrease in leptin, the hormone that regulates appetite. Adiponectin levels also increased in all groups except the one that had no changes to diet or physical activity. The changes to these hormones lead to less voracious appetites, resulting in eating less and weight loss while also providing a boost of anti-inflammation support. Hormonal regulation, as demonstrated in this study, explains why health organizations promote the combination of better nutrition and food choices with physical activity.

Finally, the link between exercise and better nutrition is that a physically active body causes cells to increase the production of proteins that help to break down antioxidants so that they can become full-fledged cancer fighters. This is just one of many facts that point to how physical activity and eating patterns work together to fight off another bout of breast cancer.

Physical Activity Improves Mood

My days as an exercise leader are behind me, yet I continue to believe, and research has shown, that moving does more than sculpt your legs or strengthen your heart. Physical activity, like dancing around the kitchen, taking a spin around the block, or doing a few squats while talking on the phone, does more than reduce recurrence risk. It enhances your mood and decreases the depression that comes with a breast cancer diagnosis.

Like a millstone around your neck, a glum mood weighs you down, preventing you from reaching the life you have imagined after cancer treatment. This is all too common among breast cancer survivors. Think back to the earlier discussion about gratitude and finding your purpose. Depression has a way of trapping you in a place where gratefulness and the desire to make lifestyle choices remain out of reach. Depression among breast cancer survivors has not gone unnoticed, and a recent study examined four ways of delivering more physical activity to survivors. Among over three hundred women, there were four groups: supervised sessions of exercise, access to an exercise facility, Fitbit monitoring, and an Active Living Every Day (ALED) program.[64] Of the four, ALED participants had the most improvement in their depressive symptoms. Why? Because this program's focus was on how to change behavior, build skills to overcome barriers, set goals, and enlist social support. Maybe it is the goal setting and pursuit that helps with the depression. But, like the experience of my weight loss group, social networks and the support that comes from them also relieve depression. Importantly, seeking out the help of trained professionals and the camaraderie of other survivors is powerful and effective. Active Living Every Day: the name alone implies a focus on more movement and less drudgery.

Move More, Worry Less

When you move more, depression decreases and you worry less, too. Better moods, less anxiety, and physical activity go hand in hand. Researchers do not understand the precise mechanisms by which physical movement impacts stress and anxiety, but they do know that several biological, as well as psychological, systems are involved.[65] Personally, I call it a "feel-good hormone." Following a bout of physical activity, focus shifts from fret to free as possibilities emerge and concerns subside. Furthermore, by changing the chemicals in the brain and reducing anxiety and worry, you diminish negative moods and emotions. Whether you choose to call it "runner's high" or an exercise boost or something else, physical activity inspires repeat performances of good self-care. You want your life back, and more movement puts you steps closer to that end.

Regardless of economic situations, race, age, stage of cancer, prior fitness level, other illness, or family responsibilities, survivors who adhere to recommended levels of physical activity have a better quality of life and less fatigue, and they avoid weight gain and feel empowered by their efforts. Further, an ongoing discussion exists affirming that participating in regular physical activity supplies you with experiences of successfully coping with worry and agitation. A satisfied feeling comes with accomplishing a twenty-minute walk around the park or lifting hand weights while watching TV. By sticking to a physical activity program, you become more successful at managing other stressors in your life and squeezing out negative thoughts. Like the ladies in my exercise classes of years back, you get satisfaction checking the box. Physical activity for today—done. You are doing whatever you can to improve your health.

… And Bolster Your Immune System

Research also confirms that exercise enhances the immune system, your body's response to injury or disease (inflammation), and blood sugar regulation or insulin resistance.[66] All these activities affect how the machinery in our cells locates, repairs, and removes damaged cells that could become cancer cells. This is much like what an anti-inflammatory eating habit does to fight cancer. Following toxic cancer treatments, regular moderate physical activity causes the body to increase the levels of immune response components, which improves how our cells look for and uncover any lingering cancer cells. And older breast cancer survivors, who often have less efficient immune function, regain better and quicker immune system function with physical activity. Like a polypill, physical movement makes it difficult for cancer cells to grow, improves mood, increases confidence, and strengthens immunity. A super medicine.

Treatment Upsets Your Balance

As if the upheaval of your life is not enough aggravation, consider that chemotherapy and hormonal therapies can affect the balance center of the inner ear, also called the vestibular system. When your balance center is affected, you are at risk for falls that can result in bone fractures. Neuropathy caused by chemotherapy further challenges your balance, especially if it is found in your feet.

A fear of falling is enough to hinder your efforts to become more active, and for good reason. Indeed, women who have received treatment for breast cancer have a 15 percent higher risk of falls compared to women who have not undergone cancer treatment.[67] In a 2011 study published in *Archives of Physical Medicine and Rehabilitation*, researchers found that of the sixty participating survivors, nearly 60 percent of them had fallen over the past year. Results of this study, which set out to identify how nerve, muscle, balance, and vision factors contribute to falls in breast cancer survivors, suggest that balance troubles in the inner ear and vision problems are connected to increased falls.[68] Muscle coordination problems and weakness, low blood counts, a change in medications, vision changes, and unintended weight loss also put you at a greater risk of falls.

A fall can derail your recovery from treatment or add to a loss of daily function, leading to more health issues. Many survivors choose to begin their physical activity regimens by first addressing balance related to treatment side effects. They often choose to do so by meeting with a physical therapist, who gives reassurance and confidence after she has assessed your abilities. That alone makes you safer.

You may ask, "Is there a set of maneuvers proven to improve balance better than others?" One study from 2019 set out to find the answer. The group of researchers compared various types of physical activities—aerobic step, balance training, resistance training, and wobble board training—and discovered that inactivity, more than a specific type of physical activity, plays a pivotal role in the processes involved in balance. Increasing your daily physical movement reduces a fall by 30–50 percent. Walk, dance, do yoga, balance on one foot for a few minutes each day, or march in place while you watch TV; the point is to become more active at whatever you can safely do.[69] Recreation centers and online programs for balance are often modified for older survivors. (See the Resources section for this chapter for more information.)

Move More to Care for Your Bones

A fall is always unwelcome, but with thinning bones, it can be catastrophic. During visits with survivors taking anti-hormonal therapies, namely aromatase inhibitors such as anastrozole and letrozole, my discussion usually turns to bone health. Usually prescribed after chemotherapy and radiation are completed, these medications effectively lower estrogen levels in the body, preventing a relapse of breast cancer. One critical side effect of this therapy is loss of bone density. Weight-bearing physical activity is recommended to preserve bone mass, and as mentioned previously, calcium supplementation from foods or supplements is often suggested too.

In the early stages, bone loss is called *osteopenia.* In more advanced stages, *osteoporosis* occurs, which means bones have developed holes, making them weak and prone to breaking. But weight-bearing movements such as using resistance bands and hand weights, as well as regular walking, strengthen bones if done consistently. Over the course of three-plus years of taking an aromatase inhibitor, I lost two bone density points on a T-score, a measurement of bone loss, in my thigh bone. I was astounded at how quickly this happened, especially since I paid close attention to performing resistance weight exercises two times per week and walking three days weekly. If I had not regularly walked and lifted weights, the bone loss could have been greater.

Joint pain, another side effect of aromatase inhibitors, prompts some survivors to consider stopping this medication. Check with your oncologist before doing so. She may remind you that these medications are effective at preventing a recurrence and that slow, gradual increases in physical movement are shown to alleviate joint pain. In some instances, she may prescribe a trial of a different formulation of the aromatase inhibitor to address joint pain.

Unique Challenges for ALL Survivors

As mentioned earlier, estrogen-positive breast cancer gets the most attention, and this is related to the fact that most breast cancer diagnoses are estrogen-positive. Research has not confirmed how physical movement impacts women with genetically driven or estrogen-negative breast cancers (such as a genetic family history of BRCA1 and BRCA2 cancers), although a 2011 study in the *Journal of Medical Oncology* presented emerging evidence to support the link between physical activity and longer survival for women with a high-risk breast cancer (a cancer that is likely to relapse or spread).[70] The women participating in this study who did regular and consistent activity were less likely to have cancer return. Getting physically active at any point and even at lower-than-recommended levels gave a better survival advantage.

More recently, in 2020, a large National Cancer Institute study added to existing proof of the link between physical activity and longer survival in women diagnosed with high-risk breast cancer. Women in this study who met the weekly physical activity guidelines both before their diagnosis and in the two years after had a 55 percent reduced chance of cancer returning and a 68 percent reduced chance of death from any cause, not just breast cancer. Interestingly, women in the study who did not meet the guidelines before diagnosis but met them at their two-year follow-up visit had a 46 percent reduced chance of recurrence and a 43 percent reduced chance of death from any cause when compared with those who did not meet physical activity recommendations either before or in the two-year follow-up.[71] The bottom line is that when you are physically active, in the greatest amount possible and at the highest level possible, it is better than nothing, regardless of whether you have an estrogen-positive, estrogen-negative, or genetically-driven type of cancer. Like the upside of improved eating patterns and modest weight loss, physical activity is another habit that affords greater good than harm.

Pain, Posture, and Qigong

Some may have pain to the point that an effort to begin physical activity will be derailed permanently. I was pleased to find that research is aiming to figure out what can be done about what doctors call persistent post-surgical pain (PPSP) and the role qigong movements may have in addressing it.[72] It is believed that PPSP affects 25–60 percent of breast cancer survivors. This kind of pain is defined as dull, burning, or aching, mostly felt in the chest, armpit, or upper arm. It often lasts more than three months after surgery and impacts mood, increases fatigue, affects sleep and daily activities, and ruins posture. Together, these side effects add up to a diminished image of ourselves.

Our body image and emotional health are intertwined, researchers believe. And breast cancer survivors are prone to a skewed body image and emotional strain after surgery. Although Jody, a fifty-nine-year-old survivor, had surgery over eight years ago, she still holds her left arm in an awkward, scrunched-up way, which is what she did for months to "protect" herself from getting bumped, especially in crowds or tight spaces. While this has not kept her from exercising, she has developed pain with certain movements of her shoulder and arms. Physical therapists possess the expertise to help in a situation such as Jody's. After breast cancer surgery, you may notice how you position your body differently in response to lingering discomfort. And it is interesting to learn how our posture and our emotional health can be impacted by long-term pain from these surgeries.

Researchers believe that PPSP has negative effects on sleep, daily living, and quality of life. A study initiated in 2022 is investigating the use of qigong to assist breast cancer survivors with both physical posture and mood. Originating in China, qigong is a mind-body exercise incorporating coordinated movements, breath training, mindfulness, and mental focus/imagery. I am hopeful that qigong can help other survivors work through prolonged pain so that they are no longer held back from other types of exercise. Results from this study will be available a few years from now.

Health Inequalities and Barriers to Movement

We all need some level of physical activity. This is easier for some to accomplish than others. Stage of cancer, treatment, age, family responsibilities, other diseases, racial disparity, economic concerns, prior fitness level, and support are different for all of us. Household budgets do not always have the funds for gym memberships, fitness classes, and an assortment of sneakers. The need for a walking partner may be the only way to safely walk in your neighborhood. Some of you may have your share of challenges that derail efforts to become more active: safety, costs, family caretaking responsibilities, and cultural standards. I cannot forget Wanda, a sixty-year-old Hispanic grandmother raising three grandchildren on a bare-bones budget. Without access to a car, Wanda rode the bus to work, leaving little time to "go for a stroll." As a member of my survivors' weight loss group, the other survivors suggested increasing her daily steps by taking an extra lap around the parking lot at work and taking a longer route after getting off the bus on her way home. Her budget did not easily afford new walking shoes or a health club membership. Living situations like Wanda's require creativity and troubleshooting.

Until recently, most activity studies have focused primarily on Caucasian women. Cancer centers are learning that minority groups have varied needs for getting more physically active. Often, it is not a lack of desire; it is a matter of safety, affordability, cultural considerations, and time. For example, a study from the National Institute on Minority Health and Health Disparities showed that Latinas favor access to a social network for support. Not surprisingly, study results suggest that this group responds well to culturally sensitive education and, at the same time, embraces the use of technology, such as smartphones, to reinforce their physical activity.[73]

Similarly, African American breast cancer survivors are less likely to engage in physical activity compared with Caucasian women. Family childcare, costs, job obligations, and distance stand in the way of survivors who wish to become more active. Furthermore, African American women often have not only more advanced diseases but are at greater risk for weight gain, diabetes, and heart problems. Side effects of treatment and complications heaped on top of these barriers move physical activity down the priority list at a time when more movement is crucial. A study from *Integrative Cancer Therapy Journal* explored how a home-based physical activity model could be used to help increase daily activity among African American breast cancer survivors. The sixteen-week program provided telephone support to help motivate women to increase activity in their homes. At the conclusion of the study, significant physical and mental improvements were noted,[74] most likely because the participants received the kind of support they needed to become successful. Guidance delivered in a language you understand and with an eye and ear on the cultural, financial, and physical limitations you have can make all the difference in whether you grab on to more activity or stay on the couch.

And of course, as we get older, greater encouragement is needed to begin physical movement due to difficulties such as cost, transportation, access, and appropriate levels of activities. If you have diabetes or heart disease on top of breast cancer, other challenges emerge. When meeting with your oncologist or a physical therapist, it is important to mention your hurdles. Access to recreation facilities and transportation is a common barrier that survivors encounter. Survivors have shared with me that being among non-survivors in community-based fitness classes can be intimidating, even embarrassing, as they struggle to keep up with the pace of the group. Proper footwear is another common hurdle. A diagnosis of diabetes with numbness in your feet, for example, requires a closer look at the footwear you choose. A wider, sturdier sole helps with neuropathy to give you better balance and "feel." There are solutions to your obstacles, and troubleshooting these during visits with your doctor or physical trainer overcomes the hindrances.

Barriers can be overcome with the right tools and approaches. With a little effort, you can access tools to help. Grabbing a partner to walk with will increase your enjoyment and your fitness. Getting your family to buy in on your physical activity plan makes it easier for you to devote yourself to your goals. After a while, you discover that a walk around the park with a friend is helping you to get your life back.

Progressive, gradual increases in physical activity lead to greater fitness, but support is critical to making this a reality. I repeatedly hear from survivors that what they want and need most to become more physically active is a plan designed specifically for their fitness level and daily schedules. Behavior change, which is what diet and exercise habits require, demands more than a handout or quick review of the recommendations for exercise, which is why getting the right amount and type of guidance is critical.

If you live in a large city, university-based cancer centers may offer home- and facility-based exercise programs for survivors. I favor finding others in your faith community, workplace, survivor support groups, or neighborhood and asking them to join you as you exercise. Your resolve to make exercise a habit is strengthened when others rely on you and you on them. Together the group solves the issues all encounter for moving more, and this alone increases your success. More movement leads to more glistening!

Around the Block or Around the Pool, You Choose

The facts in favor of physical movement may be enough to get you to order new shoes and head out the door every day for a walk or a bike ride around the block a few times after dinner. But what if that is not enough? What if you need other reasons to get out the door? Consider one more benefit of regular exercise: exposure to sunlight when exercising outside increases vitamin D levels, and this supports the cells' ability to regulate correctly and avoid the development of cancer. And, regular exercise, particularly in groups of like-minded women, offers relaxation and friendship, giving way to the enjoyment of physical activity. According to Hippocrates, walking is a woman's best medicine—it is also the most accessible. And because more footwear manufacturers are creating walking shoes with a wide base, which helps with neuropathy, it is more comfortable to get outdoors.

Modifying the amount of time and the intensity of moderate or more vigorous daily activities may be the key to your physical fitness plan. For example, if you walk from the parking lot to the storefront, an increase in your pace or a lap around the parking lot before you get back into the car are both ways to increase physical activity. Dancing around the kitchen for a minute or two longer each day will gradually increase exercise amounts. A fitness plan does not have to be complicated to be effective.

What are Moderate and Vigorous Physical Activities?

Moderate	Vigorous
• brisk walking • biking • swimming • mowing the lawn	• running • swimming laps • heavy yard work • aerobic dancing

A *low* level of physical movement includes daily activities and for some, more household chores or a trip to the mailbox may be your starting line. *Moderate* exercise means you can talk to your friend while you are moving, while *vigorous* movement makes conversation harder. What if you add a minute or two of vigorous movement to a daily walk or dancing? You may find you can do more than you thought, just not for long periods. Although no research has yet pinned down the exact dose of physical activity needed to reduce the risk of death from cancer, more activity appears to lead to better risk reduction. Long bouts of vigorous activity are not necessary. Activity at an intensity and amount for you is important. Small increases in physical activity supply notable results as you work up tolerance.

Remember, Keep it Simple.	Get Expert Support and Guidance.	Talk with Your Doctor.	Build a Plan That Works.
If you just received your diagnosis, simply find reasons to get up and move throughout the day. In survivorship years? Then begin with short bouts of movement and add on gradually as you develop strength.	Ask if your hospital or local wellness center has a cancer rehabilitation program. Certified Cancer Exercise Trainers, some physical therapists, or a member of your care team can help you design a safe physical activity program for you.	Are there limits on physical activity caused by surgery, chemotherapy, or radiation? What side effects do you have that limit some types of activity?	Keep a log of your activity, medications, fatigue (0-10), and pain. This will help you discover what works. Find an activity partner or support group to keep you motivated.

Adapted from Being Active When You Have Cancer originally published by American College of Sports Medicine.

Begin Safely, Go Slowly, Do What You Can

The hard part about adding a physical activity routine is to get started. The best place to begin is by getting clearance from your doctor, who can help you decide what types of physical activity are safe for you. She may refer you to a physical therapist with cancer rehabilitation expertise or to a program in the community designed for cancer survivors. These important steps help you avoid injury and setbacks that come with physical activity that is too strenuous. Beginning safely and slowly allows your confidence to increase while your body responds.

Experts see the benefits of physical activity done in short chunks of time spread throughout each day. According to Bob Murray, PhD, FACSM, co-author of *Food and Fitness After 50,* regular physical activity improves our "health span," or the length of time that we are healthy. Increasing the health span is possible without heavy sweating, running, or other strenuous movements. In fact, the real goal is to reduce the amount of time you sit each day while increasing the amount of time you are moving. By adopting a habit of activity breaks of *any* duration, you increase your health span. Your own plan could look like this on your first day:

Activity Breaks Chart

First Day:

Time of day	Physical activity type	Amount of time
Morning break	Walking or dancing	3 minutes
Evening break	Walking or dancing	3 minutes

A day later, your plan could look like this:

Activity Breaks Chart

Time of day	Physical activity type	Amount of time
Morning break	Walking or dancing	4 minutes
Evening break	Walking or dancing	4 minutes

By increasing the length of your activity break by one minute each day, you safely build up to a plan with three activity breaks. A week or so later, your plan is to add one more activity break and increase your walking to a faster pace:

Activity Breaks Chart

Time of day	Physical activity type	Amount of time
Morning break	Fast walking or dancing	5 minutes
Midday break	Fast walking or dancing	5 minutes
Evening break	Fast walking or dancing	5 minutes

Small but measurable and gradual increases in both time and intensity get you to the recommended thirty minutes of moderate activity on five days of the week.

Sample of 150 minutes of Weekly Physical Activity for Beginners

Day 1	Day 2	Day 3	Day 4	Day 5	Day 6	Day 7
30 minutes of walking	Rest	30 minutes of walking	30 minutes of hand weights or band resistance training	Rest	30 minutes of walking	30 minutes of stretching and balance exercise

You may feel intimidated by physical activity recommendations. Fitting in one more thing can break the delicate balance of your schedule. But moving more is medicine: it helps fight fatigue and anxiety, bolsters immune function, furnishes strength to complete chores, reduces lymphedema symptoms, and improves overall health. For the weight loss group at my cancer center, I tracked minutes of physical activity weekly for each of our participants. Only a few women in the group committed to regular exercise near the recommended levels. In fact, those who committed to regular activity were able to maintain their weight loss.

Walking toward What the Future Holds

Thankfully, survivors are living longer and better. Years ago, when I began my cancer dietitian career, survivors were asked to stop physical activity as soon as they were diagnosed. From my vantage point, telling a survivor to avoid movement and just rest sounded like an invitation to allow illness to settle in and stay. But this approach is changing quickly, and now physical movement is another way that you can feel fully alive and energized. The National Institute of Cancer believes that researchers and doctors are moving closer to that point at which they can dose exercise precisely for every survivor, just as they do with drugs. Through a presidential initiative, Kathryn Schmitz, PhD, created Moving Through Cancer, a program supported and promoted by the American College of Sports Medicine (ACSM) with the goal that all people living with cancer are assessed, advised, referred to, and engaged in appropriate exercise through their cancer journey.[75] Supporters of the program believe strongly that survivors should receive a physical activity plan geared to individual needs and abilities while receiving treatment and beyond. Granted, this is just the beginning of bringing individualized physical activity opportunities to all survivors. My hope is that one day soon, all survivors will receive the necessary education and support to meet the recommendations.

Get Expert Help

Once your doctor or physical therapist agrees it is safe for you to get more activity, do a little homework before joining a gym or recreation center. Thousands of exercise professionals out there are ready to help you, but not all fitness leaders are created equal, especially when it comes to educating, motivating, and guiding survivors. Remember, as a survivor, your needs are unique. After treatment, you need more attention than you will get in a standard community exercise class. A specialized program tailored to your limitations and strengths is best but not always available.

To illustrate how specialized classes help, consider that breast cancer survivors with extensive lymphedema may first require the expert ability of a physical therapist. A woman with numbness (neuropathy) in her feet or hands will need a set of balance exercises from a trainer with knowledge about the side effects of chemotherapy. The cancer exercise therapist (CET) is a relatively new certification for exercise professionals who wish to customize activities for survivors, and the programs created by a CET are carefully designed to meet your physical needs. Recreation centers, university exercise programs, and private gyms may employ these specialized trainers.

Like-minded survivors filling up an exercise room inspire you, and trainers with special training know how to push you safely and pull you back when needed. See the Resources section for this chapter to find a CET in your area.

Joyful Inspiration: Linda's Story

Linda, a fifty-three-year-old woman with hyperthyroidism when she was diagnosed with stage 3 breast cancer, joined my weight loss group and is a fine example of getting the help you need to get started and stay motivated. With ongoing fatigue, neuropathy in her feet and hands, and lymphedema, Linda did not feel safe embarking on a physical activity plan. Thyroid problems had resulted in weight gain over the years, and cancer treatment contributed several more pounds. With an understanding that while more physical activity did not necessarily lead to weight loss, she knew that becoming more active would help her maintain the weight she was losing through better food choices. Also, she understood that aerobic dance and weight training classes at her recreation center were out of the question. Following several visits with the cancer center physical therapists, Linda felt ready to branch out to her local recreation center for more variety and challenge. With encouragement from the weight loss group, she was determined to reclaim her health through improved food choices as well as improve her balance and endurance so she could move more.

Linda joyfully explored different ways to safely move and reported back to the group. On the advice of her physical therapy team, she began with water exercises. After several sessions of water exercises, she learned how the movements helped manage her lymphedema with fluid arm movements and encouraged others to try this activity. Without fear of falling and no need for her compression sleeve, Linda experienced how water exercise allowed her to move and stretch while also rebuilding her endurance. Water was her safety net, allowing her to move for longer and decreasing her fatigue. Always picking up tidbits of information from books and videos, Linda reported back to the group that "our lymphatic system does not have a propulsion system. It relies solely on our movement to navigate and flow through our body. This system is essential to our well-being and bodily function. It keeps our body fluid levels balanced and defends against infections." Her willingness to investigate classes and information inspired others in the group to seek out their preferred activity. I smiled while hearing her comments, as I realized she had been sold on the idea of more physical activity.

After several months of water workouts, Linda progressed to a Nia dance class, which is designed to allow participants to move without impact, using arms and legs in fluid movements. Linda found the Nia classes allowed her to move without trying to balance on one foot to change direction. Over the course of a year, she tried yoga, Pilates, qigong, and tai chi classes. Not long after, she organized a survivors' walking group that continues today. She walks four miles several times weekly using walking sticks as support.

A weight loss of more than twenty pounds helped her move better and feel better. More than anything, Linda wanted to find ways to have greater overall health. One dance with cancer is enough, she wryly shared with me. Reclaiming her health, both body and soul, required safe places where she could share her challenges, seek solutions, and have no fear of injury. Better food choices, modest weight loss, and more physical movement brought her a sense of accomplishment and the satisfaction of knowing she was doing all that she could to prevent a recurrence. As a strong proponent of the power of the combination of food and physical activity as medicine, Linda says that her quality of life has improved.

Something Is Better Than Nothing

Personally and professionally, I believe becoming more active should be at the top of your list of lifestyle changes. Of course, I favor healthy eating, but I believe moving more eventually leads to enhanced eating habits. When you feel good about your body, you have a renewed desire to fuel it with better foods. Good things come when you sweat, even if you prefer a glisten: less stress, improved confidence, greater calm, lower blood sugar and inflammation, and stronger muscles. You walk a little taller, feel good in your clothes, and like what you see in the mirror when you are more physically active. Another advantage is that modest weight loss or weight stability is often the result of physical activity. A goal of daily activity means you will not miss a dose of this powerful medicine.

Finding your own tempo, rhythm, and pace is key to making physical movement a daily routine. So is knowing how to safely begin and which styles of movement are best for you. Most of us have lingering side effects, including fatigue, pain, feet numbness, muscle weakness, and shortness of breath. And all of us can benefit from some level of physical activity, no matter how limited. A favorite saying of mine is "Something is better than nothing," which helps to frame expectations, especially if you think that physical activity involves grand plans such as a marathon, a monster-size hike, or swimming the English Channel. You and I both have something left over after treatment that keeps us from being as active as we would like. But that does not mean we cannot do more. We find movements that are best for us and ease us into moving more, and we do so gracefully. Good things come to you as you glisten.

It is tempting to believe that physical activity is a cure, a sure thing against a recurrence of cancer or other health problems, but leading experts say that physical activity is not the only factor. Physical movement is, however, an essential component in your survivorship toolbox and one that you can manage at a level you choose. Physical activity makes you shine a little more. And success with some exercise gives you the confidence you need to do more each day. And of course, even before weight loss through a calorie-reduced diet occurs, exercise directly lowers levels of excess estrogen and leptin, both of which are known to promote estrogen-positive breast cancer. Regardless of the type of breast cancer you have, I love seeing you get the satisfaction of working through the challenges of treatment side effects, and I love seeing you thrive. Physical movement affords you the confidence that you are doing whatever it takes to do more than survive. Few things are more satisfying for me than hearing you say, "I did it!"

KEY POINTS

- Women who exercise after their diagnosis have a lower risk of relapse or death from their cancer as well as less risk for other diseases.

- Physical activity and better eating patterns deliver a one-two punch against breast cancer.

- The best place to begin an exercise regimen is with your doctor. She can make referrals to physical therapists or other cancer exercise professionals to help you begin safely.

- Something is better than nothing when it comes to adding physical activity. Begin safely, use what you have, go slowly, and do what you can.

In The Pink

"Nay, I am the very pink of courtesy."

—ROMEO AND JULIET, ACT 2, SCENE 4, BY WILLIAM SHAKESPEARE

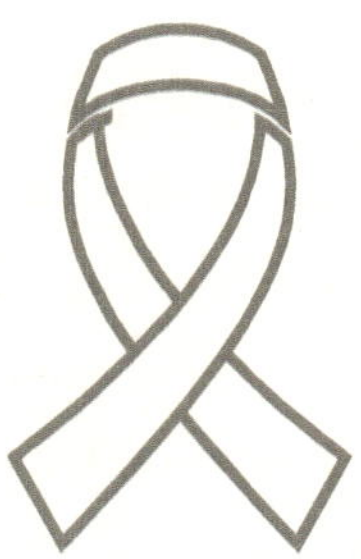

LIKE THE STROKE OF COLOR TO A CANVAS, in this chapter, you learn to apply personal changes with a tender touch. By chapter's end, you will be ready to adopt one or two new habits. This chapter gathers what you learned in previous chapters, helping you craft an eating pattern suited to your needs and ideally joining it with more physical activity.

You explored how to begin with gratitude, learning the power of optimism and walking toward your why. Then you discovered how trading old habits for better ones moves you out of your comfort zone, flexing the muscles of confidence and motivation as you adopt new health practices. The food as medicine concept dispelled the mystery of inflammation, introduced energy- and nutrient-dense food, and answered questions about making every bite count toward a healthier future. More pieces of the puzzle emerged as you considered how weight affects health risks and learned how to use food groups and eating patterns to your advantage. The chapter about glistening demonstrated how physical activity improves mood, immune function, and bone strength, and it enhances the benefits of a healthy eating pattern. Steadily, the chapters unveiled the tools needed for you to arrive at the best of health and in good spirits—to live in the pink.

In this chapter, you will:

- Review how an eating pattern designed for a lifetime improves your nutritional health and controls weight.

- Take a deeper look at food groups containing evidence-based nutrients important for breast cancer survivors.
- Discover the skills you need to adopt a new eating style.
- View a demonstration of enhancements to Kathy's meal plan (featured in chapter 4) as you learn to layer nutritional details and build an eating pattern based on your health issues, personal preferences, and nutritional goals.

Splashes of earlier ideas are scattered about in this chapter: nutrient- and energy-density, antioxidants, inflammation, and the four food groups are recognizably applied for the greater health of breast cancer survivors. Along the way are mealtime planning suggestions. All of this leads you to a healthier shade of pink.

Now What Do I Eat?

It is no surprise to me that soon after treatment, you were seeking answers to your questions about what to eat. Increasing antioxidants, specific diets, losing weight, foods to avoid or add—these are good starter topics, and some answers were revealed in earlier chapters. Recall the discussion about restrictive diets like raw, keto, and others in chapter 2. You want the weight off. Now. Treatment is over, and your desire to lose weight and eat better surfaces.

First, take a breath.

Fad diets come and go with the latest headlines or breakroom chatter. By design, fad diets are missing at least one food group: remove bread, crackers, and desserts—and you will lose weight. Diets that are missing a food group will not properly fuel your body, the body that suffered through side effects and fatigue. Fad diets often result in massive amounts of weight loss in the short term, but staying on a fad diet for the rest of your life is not feasible. You deserve better.

Several years ago, a client approached me, saying she could not understand why her hair was falling out. As it turns out, she had been following a raw diet, a vegan plan of eating fruits, vegetables, nuts, and seeds for six months, and she had lost thirty pounds. A lack of protein and other nutrients resulted in her hair loss. Following fad diets can lead to physical symptoms such as hair and muscle loss and digestive issues, specifically constipation. With various restrictions of fruits, fats, breads, and pasta, these diets can lead to fiber, vitamin, and mineral deficiencies.

Restrictive diets can be effective in the short run. Blood sugar and cholesterol levels drop and the weight peels off, but fad diets are not effective at restoring or maintaining health. In the end, nutrition experts agree that the best diet is one you can stick to for a lifetime. An eating style that does not cause symptoms of poor nutrition or lead to boredom and extreme hunger is best.

A Plan You Can Follow for Life

In "Food as Medicine," I presented a formula for healthier eating after breast cancer:

1. **Improve the quality of your eating pattern by choosing lean proteins, higher fiber from whole grains, and fruits and vegetables.**
2. **Focus on foods that are high in nutrient-density to support the health of your cells. Limit energy-dense, high-calorie foods that deliver few nutrients.**
3. **The combination of 1 and 2 will result in a modest 5–10 percent weight loss and improved nutritional health, thus lowering your risk of disease.**

For review, nutrient-dense foods are jam-packed with anti-inflammatory components like antioxidants, vitamins, and minerals, all of which give our cells the stuff needed to fight off cancer and other diseases and restore health after treatment. Broccoli, fish, lean chicken, low-fat cheese, eggs, and whole wheat bread are examples of nutrient-dense foods. Your body deserves bowls and plates containing mostly nutrient-dense foods. Energy-dense foods, also known as fun foods, such as ice cream, candy, alcohol, and fried foods, are high in saturated fat, added sugars, and calories, with few nutrients. Eaten sparingly, these foods allow room in the bowl or on the plate for nutrient-dense choices.

The Swarm of Phytonutrients

Inflammation. Oxidative stress. Free radicals. Antioxidants. Phytonutrients. Simply put, the first three in this list are bad for your health, while antioxidants and phytonutrients are helpful. Inflammation, as you learned earlier, is the protective response of your immune system, resulting in the production of oxidants, also known as free radicals or reactive oxygen species, in cells.

Examples Of Phytonutrients In Vegetables and Fruits	
Lycopene:	tomatoes, pink grapefruit, watermelon
Anthocyanins, polyphenols:	berries, grapes, unsweetened grape juice, plums
Alpha and beta-carotene:	carrots, mango, pumpkin
Beta-cryptoxanthin, flavonoids:	cantaloupe, peaches, oranges, papaya, nectarines
Lutein, Zeaxanthin:	spinach, avocado, honeydew, collard, turnip greens
Sulforaphane, indoles:	cabbage, broccoli, brussels sprouts, cauliflower
Allyl sulfides:	Leeks, onion

As a broad term for the variety of compounds produced by plants, *phytonutrients* ("phyto" is a prefix meaning "plant") are derived from fruits, vegetables, whole grains, nuts, beans, and tea. Once eaten and digested and finally inside the cells, phytonutrients become the good guys, swarming around to stamp out free radicals (the "bad guys") that appear with inflammation.

Another commonly used name for phytonutrients is phytochemicals, but this term applies to plant chemicals used for protecting plants from bugs, fungi, and other threats. While phytonutrients are not critical for keeping you alive in the same manner as vitamins and minerals, they may protect against disease and aid in the optimal function of body systems. Experts believe there are up to twenty-five thousand varieties of phytonutrients, and each one comes from different plant sources with various benefits for the body. Phytonutrients commonly showcased in magazines or headlines are carotenoids, of which there are six hundred varieties, ellagic acid found abundantly in berries, flavonoids of which there are three types, resveratrol found in red grapes and wine, sulforaphane inside broccoli and cabbage, and phytoestrogens contained in soy, flax, and sesame seeds. From this list, this chapter will go into more depth regarding carotenoids, flavonoids, sulforaphane, and phytoestrogens, as these are of particular interest for fighting breast cancer.

Powerful Plant Nutrients for Breast Cancer Survivor

Sulforaphane (Cruciferous)	Carotenoids	Flavonoids	Phyto-estrogens
arugula	apricots	beets	soybeans
broccoli	cantaloupe	cherries	flax seeds
Brussels sprouts	carrots	citrus fruits	tofu
cabbage	kale	dark berries	tempeh
cauliflower	papaya	edamame/ tofu/soy milk	dried fruit
collard greens	spinach	garlic	chickpeas
daikon cabbage	sweet potatoes	radishes	garlic
horseradish	leafy greens	red grapes/ juice	peanuts
kale	tomatoes	turnips	
wasabi	citrus	white button mushrooms	

Exactly how phytonutrients work is not clearly understood, but as a group, they fulfill a variety of tasks. They protect against oxidative stress, promote cancer cell death, alter hormone metabolism, enhance immune function, protect against environmental toxins, and promote a healthy mixture of good bacteria in the gut. A phytonutrient may be a vitamin known to enhance health processes, like how carotene found in vitamin A benefits vision or how sulforaphane found in broccoli fights cancer.[76] A comic book representation of superheroes swooping in to rescue people from an invasion from above is one way to visualize how phytonutrients work. Although this is oversimplified, just as Superman or Spider-Man arrive seemingly out of thin air to aid entire cities, phytonutrients, too, are on the lookout for bad guys, and they stand ready to remove them from the vicinity.

Popular interest in antioxidants, a subgroup of phytonutrients, arises from what is known about how this group protects against damage caused by free radicals. *Free radicals* are unstable chemicals coming from stress, toxins, drugs, the environment, and other sources, and they are capable of harming cells. The harm caused to cell structures and processes can lead to diseases like cancer or heart disease. Free radicals are naturally formed in the body as part of normal cell processes when an atom either gains or loses an electron (a small negatively charged particle in atoms).[77] Accumulating free radicals, such as occurs with inflammation, damages critical parts of cells, including deoxyribonucleic acid (DNA), protein, and cell membranes. DNA damage is believed to play a role in the development of cancer and other diseases.

Antioxidants such as vitamins A and C cancel out free radicals by seizing upon cell invaders such as toxins, drugs, and others. By attaching to an invader, antioxidants prevent damage to the cell and specifically protect DNA to maintain cell function and prevent cancer.

Can Antioxidant Supplements Help Prevent Cancer?

Perhaps you dislike vegetables or fruits and are considering getting antioxidants from a phytonutrient-containing supplement as advertised on television, on the radio, in magazines, and on social media. Buyers must be aware of phony phrases, like the ones listed in "Food as Medicine," in reference to phytonutrient supplements and the role they have in stamping out cancer. Before reaching for your pocketbook, keep in mind that the body makes some of the antioxidants needed to neutralize free radicals but relies on external sources, primarily fruits, vegetables, grains, beans, and nuts, to get the rest. For now, human studies looking at whether the use of antioxidant supplements reduces the risk of cancer presents mixed results. Still, many cancer survivors are challenged to eat five or more daily servings of fruits and vegetables, and you may reach for supplements such as the popular mixed fruit and vegetable concentrates sold in bottles and capsules.

While studies have demonstrated that these supplements do increase blood levels of important plant nutrients, especially in people who do not eat a healthful diet, there is no evidence that they reduce the risks of cancer.[78] Supplemental tabs, capsules, and concentrates are costly and not risk-free. A cautionary tale comes from a now-famous 1994 study that examined supplementing vitamin A in smokers. The study was canceled after an increased number of smokers in the study ended up with lung cancer, presumably caused by the high doses of vitamin A.[79] These study results are but one example of how more of a good thing, like a supplement, is not always a better thing. As for supplementing antioxidants and other nutrients, try food first.

Since there are over twenty-five thousand phytonutrients, many not yet well-researched, a thoughtful approach is key to optimizing the health of breast cancer survivors. Included in the discussion that follows are mentions of various phytonutrients commonly featured in the media. Specifically, for our purposes in this chapter, the spotlight shines on four with evidence backing their breast cancer-fighting capabilities: sulforaphane, carotenoids, flavonoids, and phytoestrogens. Recipes mentioned in these sections are found in the companion journal.

Sulforaphane: Learn to Love Stinky Vegetables

Cruciferous vegetables, the common name for smelly broccoli, kale, cabbage, brussels sprouts, and others, contain two plant chemicals, sulforaphane and indole, which have been studied for their anti-breast cancer effects. Sulforaphane may reduce cancer cell growth in multiple ways. First, sulforaphane disrupts the growth and division of cancer cells, and second, it promotes the death of cancer cells.[80] Future research will delve further into the potential role that sulforaphane may have used in combination with conventional drugs, such as chemotherapy or aromatase inhibitors, to further fight breast cancer. For now, piling your plate with cruciferous vegetables may be malodorous, but think about the bonus of adding them as a dose of cancer-fighting capability to mealtimes.

The ***In the Pink Plate Plan*** featured in chapter 7 follows the DGA's recommended one and a half to three and a half cups of vegetables per day, depending on calorie levels. Fewer cups for lower-calorie needs and more for higher-calorie needs. Dark green, red, and orange vegetables are important for survivors. Among these colorful groups are strong-flavored vegetables that stink more than others.

These smelly vegetables are best known for their bitterness and pairings with creamy, umami flavor additions, like Parmesan cheese and tofu, to soften strong flavors. Umami, considered the fifth taste among bitter, sour, sweet, and salty, is produced by naturally occurring glutamates found in meats, broths, tomatoes, mushrooms, and fermented cheeses.

With affordability as a bonus, cruciferous vegetables lend robust flavors and texture to meals. A bowl of broccoli, simply microwaved for a minute or two, on your plate several times per week is a simple way to fight cancer with a fork. Brussels sprouts, a favorite side, blend well with a little olive oil and a variety of spices and flavorings. A stir-fry with daikon cabbage and mixed vegetables with lean protein like chicken is a great choice for a dose of cancer-fighting cruciferous. Other recipe ideas include Asian coleslaw, collard green gumbo with ham hock, and easy roasted brussels sprouts (see the companion journal or your own recipe sources).

Carotenoids: Humble Carrots

Carrots are familiar and inexpensive vegetables packed in lunch boxes and shredded over salads. They are full of a phytonutrient called *carotenoids*, a form of vitamin A. Hues of orange and red from carotene give carrots and pumpkin their flavor and colors. There are five types of carotenoids: alpha- and beta-carotene, beta-cryptoxanthin, lutein, zeaxanthin, and lycopene, most of which are orange or yellow. Carotenoids are also found in onions, garlic, scallions, deep green vegetables like kale and spinach, corn, eggs, and citrus fruits. Studies show that women who regularly eat carotenoid-rich foods have less breast cancer risk, and the benefit applies regardless of estrogen-positive or estrogen-negative breast cancer.[81]

The affordability and variety of flavors in the carotenoid group add to their appeal. For plenty of carotenes, the In the Pink Plate Plan recommends three cups of red-orange vegetables and one cup of dark green vegetables weekly for the 1,500-calorie level. Spinach and kale, plus papaya and cantaloupe, are affordable in season and versatile in varied cooking styles. Carotenes are best absorbed through a source of fat. As an example, lycopene, a carotene found in tomatoes, is best absorbed with a drizzle of olive oil and garlic. Ideas for carotene-rich recipes are pumpkin muffins, pumpkin mac and cheese, and spring stir-fry with chicken.

Flavonoids: Natural Aromatase Inhibitors

Sulforaphane and carotenoids appear mostly in vegetables, but flavorful flavonoid, another phytonutrient, is found in a wide variety of both fruits and vegetables. With eight different flavonoid types—anthocyanins, lignans, limonene, phytic acid, proanthocyanidins, phenols, phytoestrogens, and plant stanols and sterols—this group conducts a variety of activities in the body. Because most fruits and vegetables contain more than one type of flavonoid, you get better variety by mixing and matching your daily servings.

Aromatase inhibitors such as anastrozole, letrozole, and exemestane are specially formulated to decrease estrogen and thereby stop the growth and spread of breast cancer cells. As effective as these aromatase inhibitors are for treating estrogen-positive breast cancer, researchers are studying the possibilities of natural aromatase inhibitors as an alternative or perhaps an addition to the prescription forms due to the undesirable side effects of these anti-hormonal drugs.

There are many flavonoids, so nailing down one or two that work best as a natural aromatase inhibitor is going to take a long time. An older study identified white button mushrooms and red grapes as containing the greatest concentration of natural aromatase inhibitors, but more recent reviews of naturally occurring aromatase inhibitors suggest that much remains to be understood about which foods are the best sources.[82] This means you can hold off on heaping your plate with white button mushrooms and red grapes until more is understood.

Instead, consume a wide variety of fruits and vegetables to get the greatest array of flavonoids possible. Fruits and vegetables high in flavonoids include berries of all types, red grapes, flax seed, rye grains, citrus fruits, cocoa, cinnamon, apples, parsley, sweet potatoes, leafy greens, citrus fruits, tomatoes, carrots, cranberries, pears, cucumbers, soybeans, and squash. Use recipes such as a fruit and yogurt breakfast shake, turkey and cucumber sandwich, Cobb salad with pears, and nectarine and raspberry cobbler found in the journal, or similar ones in your files, to increase flavonoid intake.

What would a registered dietitian say?

Eating too many fruits dampens efforts to lose weight. Although healthful, fruit has more sugar and, therefore, calories, than veggies. Go for more servings of vegetables and fewer servings of fruits.

Granny Was Right, Eat Your Fiber

An apple is an ordinary fruit, but hidden within the golden flesh is soluble fiber acting like a sponge to absorb excess estrogen and whisk it away to be eliminated in waste. In this way, *soluble fiber*, the kind that makes you feel fuller for longer, found in apples, unsweetened applesauce, potatoes (inner flesh), uncooked oats, muesli, beans, unripe bananas, barley, quinoa, brown rice, and lentils, may decrease the risk of estrogen-positive breast cancer.[83] *Insoluble fiber*, found in wheat and corn bran and many vegetables, plays a role in breast cancer risk, too. By putting together the results of many studies, experts found that consuming high fiber, both insoluble and soluble forms, decrease the risks of both premenopausal and postmenopausal breast cancers.[84]

Several biological processes may explain the beneficial effects of dietary fiber on breast cancer risk. Remember how inflammation involves glucose and insulin? Fiber may decrease the risk of breast cancer by controlling glucose and insulin, reducing inflammation. Overall, these findings support the ACS dietary guidelines to consume foods rich in total fiber, including fruits, vegetables, and whole grains. Banana overnight oats, barley jambalaya, and apple wedges with pumpkin almond butter recipes in the journal contain estrogen-absorbing soluble fiber. Adding one or two of these each week helps manage estrogen levels.

Great Grains

Reasonably balancing whole and refined grains is important as this impacts the quality of your eating style. With a desire for great flavor and mouthfeel, you and I understand that refined or processed grains taste good and have a satisfying bite. Processed grains are also less expensive. Processed, refined grains are deliciously tempting, and a tight food budget may not afford expensive ancient whole grains like quinoa, farro, spelt, or amaranth. But choosing whole wheat bread over white bread and brown rice instead of white is a great way to increase your whole grains and fiber without blowing your budget.

The In the Pink Plate Plan recommends four to nine ounces of total grains *daily*, depending on calorie needs. A one-ounce serving equals:

- one slice of bread
- one cup of ready-to-eat cereal
- a small tortilla
- three cups of popcorn
- a half cup of cooked rice, pasta, or hot cereal

As a reminder from "Puzzle Pieces," between a quarter and half of this recommendation is whole grains, roughly two to four ounces per day for many women, providing antioxidants, B vitamins, and fiber. And, to get much-needed iron and folate from grains, one to two ounces of daily grains should be refined.

A gentle nudge in the right direction is to replace refined grain foods with more whole grain forms. This one simple change, done over a week or two, will go a long way toward managing cravings, keeping hunger at bay, supporting cell health, and warding off inflammation. Whole grains contain insoluble fiber, help the hardworking gastrointestinal system, and absorb toxins, which are then eliminated in the feces (I know, gross, but this is important).

Finally, incorporating grains into meals should be simple and not empty your pocketbook. Apple pistachio crisp, mashed avocado toast, and oatmeal pancakes are inexpensive, easy ways of getting whole grains. Another useful hack to balance processed and whole grains is using one slice of whole grain and one slice of white bread to make a sandwich. Best of both grain worlds.

Phytoestrogens: Soy, Here We Go Again

Evidence suggests moderate amounts of soy foods, nuts, and seeds fit into an overall healthy eating pattern. They are high in protein and fiber, healthy monounsaturated and polyunsaturated fats, as well as good sources of vitamin E, magnesium, phosphorus, and copper. Due to the nutrient-dense properties of nuts and seeds, with proper portion sizes, they are good stand-ins for croutons on salad or sprinkled on top of toast, cereals, and soups.

But as for soy, part of the protein foods group, survivors like you ask if it is safe and protective or if it should be avoided. This section seeks to provide answers to these questions. Soy has had a tarnished reputation for decades, in part because experts presented theories of how isoflavones, more famously known as phytoestrogens, mimic human estrogen and potentially increase estrogen levels, thereby increasing the risk of breast cancer in women who regularly eat soy foods. But worries stemming from a possible similarity between soy phytoestrogens and female estrogen in humans have been quelled with a greater understanding of the potency of isoflavones. The estrogen activity of isoflavones in soy and other plant foods ranges from a mere hundredth to a thousandth of the power of human female estrogen.[85] Researchers have expressed concern about how phytoestrogens, with a chemical structure like human estrogen, may bind to human estrogen receptors. Over the past few decades, many studies have been conducted with cells and animals (rodents), and the findings do not demonstrate the same effects in humans.[86]

Science has since proven that isoflavones have protective properties for heart health, diabetes, and cancer, and so after years of study, whole soy foods like tofu, soy milk, and edamame are considered safe for breast cancer survivors. Some nutrition scientists believe that isoflavones in soy play a beneficial role against cancer. Isoflavones may block the most potent forms of estrogen in the blood, hinting at the possibility that soy may be protective against estrogen-positive breast cancer. Isoflavones aid in the repair of DNA, prevent the growth of tumors, and have antioxidant, anti-inflammatory, and cancer-fighting elements. This plant nutrient also helps immune health and brain function. Also of interest, isoflavones reduce hot flashes, lessen the loss of bone density in the spine, assist with blood pressure during early menopause, and improve blood sugar control. For a protein food so surrounded by controversy, soy carries a fine pedigree as a healthy food. Researchers also think it is possible that some women derive more benefits from soy than others based on individual differences in digestion and absorption from one body to another.[87]

Today, the message about soy and breast cancer has shifted away from fears that soy foods increase the risk of estrogen-positive breast cancer or threaten poor outcomes after diagnosis. Now, based on so many studies about soy, leading cancer organizations have declared that breast cancer survivors can safely consume up to three servings of whole soy foods per day.[88] A serving of whole soy foods is one cup of soy milk, a half cup of edamame, or an ounce of tofu. Soy is high in protein and fiber and low in fat, making it a fine choice as a low-fat protein and a nutrient-dense food!

Whole Soy Foods and Serving Sizes

Whole Soy Foods	Serving
Tofu	1/3 cup
Soy	1 cup
Edamame	1/2 cup
Soy Nuts	1/4 cup

Wait, There Is More: Lignans

Another phytoestrogen, lignans, is found in flax seeds, rye, some vegetables, various seeds and nuts, lentils, and triticale, as well as in broccoli, cauliflower, and carrots. Lignans have shared in soy's tarnished reputation, although to a lesser degree. Like soy, lignans boost immune function, contribute to heart health, and block hormone-related cancers. Several studies have provided encouraging evidence of lignans' protective role against breast cancer, but it is not clear if the benefit extends to either or both estrogen-positive and estrogen-negative breast cancer.[89] Much like soy, lignans offer other health benefits and are safe for survivors, though questions remain as to whether they are protective specifically against breast cancer.

Confidently enjoy whole soy and lignans in meatless meals. Lignans are found in journal recipes such as Moroccan lentil stew with butternut squash and bulgur chickpea salad, which are also high in fiber. The rich sauce and flavors in the stew and the chewiness of the chickpeas in the salad are two of my favorite ways to get lignans. Grinding the flax seeds makes the nutrients more absorbable, and you can sprinkle them on yogurt and cereals or mix them in muffins.

Bone Up on Calcium

Osteopenia and osteoporosis, discussed in "Glisten," are true threats for survivors. And if an aromatase inhibitor is included in your list of medications these days, you are aware of the risks of bone thinning linked to this anti-hormonal medication. Calcium strengthens bones and, as such, is critical for bone health. For this reason, getting calcium from foods requires you to bone up by concentrating on two to three daily dairy foods.

A glass of low-fat milk or yogurt included with each meal helps meet the recommendation of 1,200 milligrams of calcium per day for women fifty-one to seventy years old. Most dairy sources contain 250–300 milligrams per serving, which suggests you need four dairy foods per day. A balanced eating pattern from all the food groups delivers an additional three hundred milligrams of calcium found in other foods, such as broccoli, almonds, leafy greens, and canned salmon. So, you aim for two to three dairy servings to meet the recommended 1,200 milligrams. Dairy milk is fortified with vitamin D, which is necessary for the absorption of calcium. Other sources of vitamin D include salmon, sardines, mushrooms, and egg yolks.

For several years, I tried diligently to eat three dairy foods per day, but after repeatedly falling short of the recommended 1,200 milligrams, I decided to supplement half of my calcium needs. For best absorption, calcium supplements are taken with food and, if supplementing the full 1,200 milligrams daily, divide the supplements into two parts. Check with your doctor before starting calcium supplements, especially if you have a history of heart issues, as calcium can aggravate irregularities of the heart function. A tool to assess your need for a calcium supplement is available in the Resources section and accompanying journal.

Rummage for Oils Like a Cavewoman

Many years ago, when your ancestors lived in caves and foraged for food, they consumed a correct balance of oils from fish, nuts, and seeds. Their diets were much higher in essential omega-3 fatty acids and lower in omega-6 and omega-9 fatty acids. Today, people eat the opposite: too much omega-6 and omega-9 and not enough omega-3. While omega-3 fatty acids reduce inflammation, omega-6 and omega-9 fatty acids tend to increase it, especially when an imbalance exists between the three types. Cavewomen did not know it, but the human body is incapable of producing omega-3 and omega-6 fatty acids, which is why they are essential, and you must get them from food. How times have changed, and what came naturally for cavewomen is today cloaked in mystery.

A visit to the oil or margarine aisle of a grocery store makes it easy to see why it is hard to identify optimal choices. Labels with words like saturated, monounsaturated (MUFAs), and polyunsaturated (PUFAs) fatty acids, plus omega-3, -6, and -9 fatty acids, are hard to understand. Here's a quick lesson to distinguish saturated, monounsaturated, and polyunsaturated fatty acids:

- Structurally, fatty acids are identified by the location and number of double bonds on a carbon chain.
- Saturated fatty acids are long carbon chains with no double bonds and are characterized by being solid at room temperature, like butter and bacon fat.

- Monounsaturated fatty acids (MUFAs), found in olive and avocado oils, have one double bond and are liquid at room temperature. Omega-9 fatty acids are monounsaturated with one double bond.

- Polyunsaturated fatty acids (PUFAs) contained in, for example, flax, walnut, canola, and rapeseed oils, have two or more double bonds and are liquid at room temperature. Omega-3 and omega-6 fatty acids are polyunsaturated with two or more double bonds.

- Fats that are liquid at room temperature are nutritionally desirable. Nutritionally unfavorable saturated fats are contained in meat, whole milk, butter, coconut oil, and bacon; these foods are solid at room temperature, while olive oil, a monounsaturated fatty acid, remains fluid. Saturated fats can cause problems with your cholesterol levels, which may increase risks for heart disease. Replacing foods that are high in saturated fat with healthier options can lower the risk of heart disease.[90]

Omega-3 fatty acids, made up of EPA (eicosapentaenoic acid) and DHA (docosahexaenoic acid), are considered polyunsaturated and are found in walnuts, flax seeds, and seafood. Because there are few omega-3 foods, getting enough of them requires dedication and planning. Soybean, rapeseed, corn, and canola oils, plus egg yolks, contain omega-6; these are the oils that Americans eat most often and in higher than recommended amounts. Omega-9 is found in the fruits and oils of avocados and olives.

Different fatty acids are desirable for different uses and flavors. Walnut oil is light and tasty in salad dressing mixtures, and olive oil pairs well with chicken dishes and marinara sauces. All the omegas are anti-inflammatory; it is the balance in favor of more omega-3 fatty acids that curbs risks for inflammatory diseases. The In the Pink Plate Plan prioritizes omega-3-rich foods for the anti-inflammatory boost against breast cancer recurrence and other diseases.

The Omegas - A Balancing Act

Omega-3s: Polyunsaturated (PUFAs)	Omega-6s: Polyunsaturated (PUFAs)	Omega-9s: Monounsaturated (MUFAs)
Eat More: Ground flax seeds, flax seed oil, walnuts, walnut oil, omega-3 fatty acid fish oil supplements, seafood (salmon, tuna)	**Balance:** Coconut oil, grapeseed oil, macadamia nuts, macadamia oil, egg yolks, soybean oil, corn oil, canola oil	**Balance:** Avocados, avocado oil, olives and olive oil, walnuts,
LIMIT • **TRANS FATS:** Strictly limit shortening and partially hydrogenated vegetable oils. • **SATURATED FATS:** Strictly limit butter, bacon, lard, sausage, whole milk/ice cream/cheese, deli meats, and heavily marbled animal meats.		

Higher intakes of food sources with omega-3 fatty acids have demonstrated a 25 percent reduction in the risk of recurrence and death in women with early-stage breast cancer. Omega-3 fatty acids have a role in reducing bone loss while also assisting with bone pain associated with these medications. Particularly in women who have received chemotherapy as part of their treatment, omega-3 fatty acids are believed to support muscle health while also preventing weight gain. Finally, these fatty acids are connected to improving attention, processing speed, immediate recall, learning, and memory in persons with impairment due to chemotherapy, also known as "chemo brain."[91]

The fats in tropical plants, such as coconut oil, palm kernel oil, and palm oil, are not included in the oils category because they contain a higher percentage of saturated fat than other oils. These three oils are often hydrogenated, a whipping process that alters the structure of the oil to extend shelf life. Hydrogenated oils are solid at room temperature and undesirable because of their effects on cholesterol levels. Bakery goods and packaged snack foods may contain hydrogenated oils. Cavewomen may not have had much choice, but in modern times, you know some oils are better than others.

Catch On to Eating Fish

Taste, cost, preparation—there are many reasons why you choose not to eat fish, but tuna, salmon, and anchovies are among the few foods with omega-3 fatty acids. Because of a need to balance oils, I encourage giving fish a try and prioritizing two servings weekly. Salmon, a common seafood choice for omega-3 fatty acids, comes in two varieties: farm-raised and wild-caught. Those that are farm-raised receive processed fish feed, and wild-caught eat wild invertebrates. Nutrient-wise, wild-caught are similar in protein content to farm-raised, slightly higher in calcium but lower in fat. Generally, wild-caught salmon are three to four times more costly than farm-raised. My twice-weekly preference for frozen wild-caught salmon, Chinook or Atlantic, cooks in twelve to twenty minutes in the oven. But I have also been known to eat and cook with farm-raised varieties too. If eating out, consider ordering salmon instead of meats to avoid high saturated fat from meats while getting a dose of omega-3 fatty acids.

More research will follow in years to come, but for now, the In the Pink Plate Plan and the DGA recommend two four-ounce servings of fish weekly, or eight ounces total. Good sources are salmon and tuna, and both are available in most regions of the US. Canned tuna is affordable and versatile on a sandwich or in salads. Although in recent years, tuna fish has received more scrutiny due to mercury levels, for now, the caution about mercury levels in tuna applies largely to pregnant women. Albacore has slightly higher mercury levels than light tuna, so buy canned light tuna in water for a quick lunch with whole grain crackers, and canned salmon for salmon burgers.

Fresh, frozen, or canned salmon—all three forms afford your heart, bones, and brain similar doses of these vital fatty acids. Not sure how to get more omega-3s? Do you like tuna salad sandwiches? Anchovies on crackers? If yes, you like fish enough to make it part of your eating choices.

Top 5 Fish Sources of Omega-3 Fatty Acids		
Salmon (Atlantic)	4 ounces	2,400 mg
Herring	4 ounces	2,290 mg
Mackerel	4 ounces	2,060 mg
Salmon (Chinook)	4 ounces	1,940 mg
Whitefish	4 ounces	1,830 mg

Start catching on to fish by adding it once weekly, with the goal of eating two times per week to get closer to the In the Pink Plate Plan recommendations.

One final note: walnuts and flax seeds/oil are popularly marketed as sources of omega-3 fatty acids. And while this claim is partially true, often left out of the walnut marketing strategy is any mention of the conversion process the body undergoes to convert the alpha-linolenic acids in the nuts to omega-3 fatty acids. Choices of foods rich in omega-3 fatty acids are limited, and if fish and walnuts are not favorites, ask your doctor about supplemental forms of omega-3 fatty acids.

The 85-15 Way Each Day

Treating yourself to a favorite splurge is part of a healthy eating pattern and a signal to your brain that these foods are, in fact, allowed in small amounts. Remember that eating patterns are not what you eat on just one day; they encompass the food choices made over days, weeks, months, and even years.

In fact, small indulgences daily can prevent the abandonment of healthy eating habits. In the long term, small rewards help with weight stability and modest weight loss.

One way to view how treats fit into your daily pattern is shown in the 85-15 diagram. Total calories for the day, consisting of nutrient-dense foods from the main groups, is represented by the larger 85 percent circle. What remains is the thin, dark outer 15 percent slice, signifying the calories that remain for small servings of energy-dense, decadent foods like ice cream, a fruit cobbler, or cheese and crackers. For a 1,500-calorie plan, 225 calories are left for small indulgences; for an 1,800-calorie plan, 270 calories are left over after eating from the nutrient-dense food groups. The fruit bar on the cover of this book represents my near-daily indulgence of eating a 120-calorie fruit bar. These frozen bars appease my craving for sweets, preventing a bigger indulgence later.

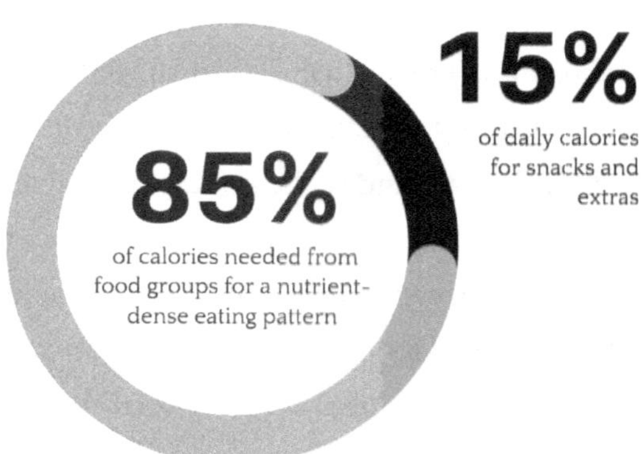

Adapted from Dietary Guidelines for Americans, 2020-2025, US Department of Agriculture and US Department of Health and Human Services, 9th Edition, December 2020.

As you have seen, there is little room for the extras, particularly as we age. The onset of menopause, either forced by treatment or naturally, plays a role in how our metabolism becomes "thrifty." As the years advance, weight gain appears easily, while shedding extra weight is extraordinarily frustrating. But prolonged deprivation from your favorite fun or junk foods sets you up for going overboard at some point, while a daily practice of saving those leftover calories for an indulgence is smart eating. A key to practicing the 85-15 way every day centers around sticking to sensible amounts of your favorite daily treats. The next chapter, "A Brighter Shade of Pink," displays the In the Pink Plate Plan with representation of the 15 percent, the outer circle in a graphic chart.

Never Starving, Never Stuffed

Working to preserve a favorite treat requires sacrifice and discipline. And a mental shift toward consuming calories aligning with your needs fundamentally alters your approach to daily meals and snacks. While embracing a little food spree each day does not come easy to those viewing a food treat as "bad," a bit of extravagance lends satisfaction, which helps you stay on track. This is one good reason in favor of a habit of tracking your food intake for sixty-six days. Doing so, as you learned in "Trade Old Habits for Better Ones," helps you reserve these few calories for a reward, much like a household budget allows for a little lavishness.

A favorite phrase of mine, "never starving, never stuffed," is a reminder to practice mindfulness around the amount of food you eat compared to the amount you need; this goes back to practicing correct portion sizes. Another way to practice this is to eat until you are 80 percent full, avoiding both hunger and going overboard. Getting too hungry carries a risk of overeating later in the day (or the middle of the night!), and overeating is more than just uncomfortable. Done consistently, eating too little or overeating undermines your efforts to pare down or keep a healthy weight and avoid health problems.

All-or-Nothing Thinking

Many people adopting a new routine fall prey to all-or-nothing thinking. This means that when you think you have already blown it, why not give in and drop this scheme to eat better or attend yoga class entirely?

A reminder: progress, not perfection. Plaster this phrase on the refrigerator, on your steering wheel, on the mirror, or on the counter. The first weeks of a new routine are brutal as your mind and body adjust to a lower amount of energy from food or push through sore muscles. Upon embarking on your new eating pattern, you experience uncomfortable hunger and your brain begins to tell you this is impossible and chides you with a remark about getting all the changes 100 percent correct or quitting. Remember, there is no such thing as a wellness garage. The process of adopting new routines, ideally, resembles the soft strokes of a feather on canvas rather than the loud clank of a wrench on steel.

Life happens. Be ready to talk back to your brain as you learned in "Trade Old Habits for Better Ones," telling it that you can acquire a new pattern, build new pathways, and signal for a new habit. You *can* do things differently, though getting there takes time and practice. Tackling the grumblings in your belly is a good place to start.

Ways to Address Uncomfortable Hunger and Stick to Your Strategy:

- Have a ready source of lean protein or high-fiber foods for times when hunger strikes. Nonfat Greek yogurt, low-fat cheese sticks, carrot sticks, an apple, or a kid-size protein bar can stave off hunger.
- Drink lots of water. Thirst is sometimes confused with hunger.
- At social gatherings, follow a Two Bite Rule. Take two bites of cheesecake/pizza/ice cream/cheese dip and be done. Your brain will have been informed that you tasted something yummy, and the taste was enough to satisfy.

- Read the menu before you arrive at a restaurant and choose appetizers, entrees, and side dishes that match up best with your eating pattern. This one habit will prevent you from falling into the temptation to order high-calorie foods like others around the table are doing.
- Make a weekly menu and create a shopping list that corresponds with the meals on the menu. This keeps you from going off the list and saves money as you avoid daily trips to the store when you are inclined to buy extra things.
- Gather cookbooks and recipes with ingredients that align with nutrient guidelines.
- Resist the chatter about the latest dessert or casserole hack on social media. While delicious, recipes that pop up may not align with your goals.

These simple tasks prepare you to avoid hunger pangs, dodge the social pressure to eat more, and help you stick to your eating plans.

What would a registered dietitian say?

All-or-nothing thinking means a survivor sees only two choices: all or nothing, with no middle option. This thinking style gets in the way of sticking to new lifestyle choices. The middle option, a balance between all and nothing, is best.

The Push-Pull of Reaching Your Goals

Practicing patience is not passive; instead, it actively requires you to set aside current behaviors and decide what the next steps will be. It involves goals that begin with hope and are then fueled by the confidence that comes from regularly pulling back, examining what works and what does not, and then pushing forward with a reinforced approach. This is the part you do within your mind—setting a daily intention to continue and pushing through temptation, distraction, and frustration. But another less anticipated test of your patience may come from your social circle.

A push against your healthier habit from family, friends, co-workers, and neighbors may be a tussle you did not anticipate. Your social circle may attempt to derail your endeavor to establish new routines. Your efforts to lose weight, eat more vegetables, drink less alcohol, and take a morning walk—each of these changes threatens the balance in your relationships.

Sabotage, as discussed in chapter 2, appears when a friend remarks that because you no longer eat fast food, you are not the lunchmate you once were. Or a news headline suggesting a fad diet for quick weight loss creates doubts about your new, improved approach to eating. Revisiting your why or purpose for making lifestyle changes will reinforce your resolve to overcome these social pressures.

Kathy, whom you met in "Puzzle Pieces," strategically placed sticky notes around her home to remind her of her promise to get healthier for her granddaughter, and Linda, introduced in "Glisten," tried several types of physical activity before moving to more difficult ones as her strength improved. Determined, Kathy and Linda set goals and patiently incorporated reminders or tried new ways to reach them.

Overcoming the pushback arises from having honest conversations with husbands or partners, family members, or co-workers, and then setting boundaries and relying on nutritional truth over lies. Create ways to deflect negative remarks or decline requests that wreck your plans. Use your newfound knowledge about food as medicine again and again to check how well you are doing. First, choose impactful changes, like eating the recommended cups of vegetables per day or two suggested weekly servings of salmon or tuna. Or begin with two five-minute activity bouts, working your way to thirty minutes a day over several days or weeks.

Nudge new lifestyle choices around the table like puzzle pieces, locking in each piece while designing your plan for a healthier life. Each time you make a grocery list, create a meal, or consider healthier options while eating out, your goals are more within your reach. It will take a stretch of time to get it like you want it, enjoying the fruits (and vegetables!) of your labor at the very top—the pinnacle—of your health. You are in the pink.

KEY POINTS

- An eating pattern you can follow for life improves nutritional health and controls weight.

- Because they are high in antioxidants and other plant properties, dark green and red/orange vegetables, along with fruits, are priority food groups for breast cancer survivors.

- Sulforaphane, carotenoids, flavonoids, and phytoestrogens are important phytonutrients with breast cancer-fighting properties.

- Breast cancer survivors can safely eat up to three servings of whole soy foods daily.

- Bone health is best preserved with three servings of dairy foods each day.

- Two servings of tuna or salmon each week provide inflammation-reducing omega-3 fatty acids.

- Eating patterns help you achieve feelings of never starving, never stuffed.

CHAPTER 7

A Brighter Shade Of Pink: In The Pink Plate Plan

"I gave to pink, the nerve of the red,
a neon pink, an unreal pink."

—ELSA SCHIAPARELLI

Your Survivorship Plan: It's Personal

The early days of my cancer experience were tinged in a fog of gray, signaling how quiet and personal this experience was for me. Over the years, though, I have gradually emerged from the haziness of those first days of my diagnosis, becoming more secure and fully fledged with acceptance of my cancer. My preference for different shades of pink has been altered; at one time, I favored a soft, whispery pink. Today, I am emboldened to wear louder, passionate shades of bubblegum and magenta, expressing my poise and confidence. As I write this, I am approaching a decade of after-breast-cancer life. Although I have had nearly ten years of clean mammograms, my lab work results reveal the very tendencies among survivors toward heart disease and diabetes presented in this book. These are like the emotional tentacles of cancer occasionally reaching in, reminding me that adherence to rock-solid routines, such as daily walks, avoiding alcohol, and sticking to my eating plan even though it is Thanksgiving, is best for me. Way back in 2014, I did not appreciate how the struggle to maintain health would cling to me like superglue, but time tells me this is my forever challenge.

Still, knowing what I know about enduring diabetes or heart disease atop my survivorship of cancer, I am unwilling to pay the price for letting healthier habits lapse ever again. All I want is a fighting chance to live the healthiest life possible. And so, old routines are now abandoned in favor of those that serve me better, but not without tempering my long-held tendency to use a hammer to create changes. A gentler touch and softer voice now occupy that place inside me that once told me to get on with it, make it so, do whatever it takes to make it happen, and seize the moments. I am done with that. After all, I am a survivor of the brightest, most unreal shade of pink.

After the completion of active treatment, your physician or nurse, with good intentions, hands you a Survivorship Care Plan. This document summarizes the care you received while hopefully igniting in you a desire to replace old habits with better ones, the "teachable moment," as it were. Doctors, nurses, and dietitians sincerely wish survivors to have healthier, longer lives, but to date, once the Survivorship Care Plan is in your possession, ongoing guidance to answer lingering questions and concerns may be minimal and inadequate. In fact, a large clinical trial demonstrated that most survivors would change behaviors for a short time, but the benefits of the education do not last long.[92] Supportive guidance, over months to years, is what is required.

Disappointment settled inside me the day I received my own Survivorship Care Plan from the nurse navigator. As she reviewed my treatments and lifestyle recommendations, I felt cheated, as I had expected something more personal about me and my needs. I wrote *In the Pink* to deliver just that: a personalized survivorship plan for you and many others.

Culminating in this chapter are the guiding principles from earlier chapters, joined together in the In the Pink Plate Plan, fashioned just for you. In this chapter, you will:

- Explore how altering an eating style over time leads to small but important changes.
- Understand how the In the Pink Plate Plan offers you a template of calorie levels, food groups in recommended amounts, and an emphasis on the seven categories deserving nutritional priority.
- Review individual topics such as budget, culture, and family and how these factors influence the formation of your eating pattern.

Until this chapter, food topics have been propped up, as though on display, for you to study. In this final chapter, you try your hand at applying what you have learned. Like an artist with an idea for a painting, you have an idea about which areas of your current eating habits could use a splash of color or which areas could disappear with a finely applied layer of black paint to obliterate them. As an eating pattern, not a diet, the In the Pink Plate Plan suggests a deliberately unrushed embrace of one food group at a time. Small, measured, delicately applied changes spread out over weeks, months, and even a year bring your eating style closer to recommendations.

Survivorship Nutrition: Art and Science

In "Trade Old Habits for Better Ones," you learned that there is no such thing as a drive-through wellness garage. I often tease that if I could wave a magic wand over you and set all your health concerns straight, I would not need to write this book. My work with Kathy demonstrated how art and science are used to construct nutritional care plans and to build upon these plans as survivors use them, reject them, or require more guidance. So much more than a list of foods, calorie levels, and food tips, her nutrition plan probed her emotional state, physical activity limitations, and previous diets—all intended to help her set realistic and personalized goals.

Kathy's Nutrition Care Plan Follow Up Visits

<table>
<tr><td colspan="4" align="center">KATHY'S NUTRITIONAL CARE PLAN: Follow Up Visits 1-4</td></tr>
<tr>
<td>Daily calorie range for weight loss:</td>
<td>1,600 – 1,800</td>
<td>Recommended Eating Pattern</td>
<td>Heart healthy vegetarian-Mediterranean-style</td>
</tr>
<tr>
<td>Goals</td>
<td colspan="3">
1. Eat at home to reduce sodium. Do not buy frozen pizzas and dinners with more than 500 milligrams of sodium. Label reading to help stay within 1,500–2,300 milligrams.
2. Vegetarian, heart-healthy food choices. Eating excess portions of processed refined grain pasta. Reviewed portions, suggested switch to whole wheat pasta. Eating lots of cheese on her pasta, so I suggested she cut down on this by 50% to decrease saturated fat.
3. Vegetarian Food Pyramid graphic reviewed to show anti-inflammatory foods in this pattern.
4. 4. Food records show too few dark green and red/orange vegetables, prefers grapes, other fruits. Educated for recommended 2 cups vegetables per day and one and one half cups dark green and four cups red/orange vegetables weekly. Food choices are low in B12, iron, and zinc and recommended asking her doctor about taking supplements.
5. Kathy likes tuna, dislikes salmon. Educated her about the benefit of adding fish to her vegetarian pattern for omega-3 fatty acids. She will think about it.
6. Most of Kathy's calcium comes from cheese estimated at 800 milligrams of calcium/day. Suggested a switch to low-fat cheese and add low-fat yogurt to lunch and dinner. She needs another 400 milligrams to meet the recommended amounts. Permission needed from heart doctor to take a calcium supplement.
</td>
</tr>
<tr>
<td>Materials Provided to Support</td>
<td colspan="3">
1. 1,400-calorie In the Pink Plate Plan
2. Sodium Content in Foods, How to Reduce Sodium from American Heart Association.
3. Vegetarian-Mediterranean food pyramid and resources reviewed.
4. Show her the Whole Grain Stamp to help identify whole grain pasta.
5. The Omegas: A Balancing Act reviewed, as well as Top Five Sources of Omega-3 Fatty Acids
6. List of high-calcium foods
</td>
</tr>
</table>

Launching Kathy's nutrition plan began with an account of her emotions, feelings, and highest motivators. Overwhelmed by fatigue and heart problems, Kathy felt that big changes to her eating habits were too big of an ask. Accordingly, in follow-up visits, Kathy and I expanded upon the original nutrition care plan with an eye on her feelings, low energy, and heart issues.

Careful attention to her heart problems was first and foremost and began with an emphasis on tips to reduce salt. She also had concerns about weight control, coupled with a desire for satisfied comfort with her foods. For both practical and emotional reasons, Kathy set a goal to maintain her weight, with an eye on improving energy levels that allowed for the enjoyment of her grandchildren. Together we agreed on a range of 1,600 to 1,700 calories per day to decrease hunger and maintain her weight. Kathy's endurance for regular physical activity was limited due to heart problems and neuropathy in her feet, leaving few safe, enjoyable activity choices. As such, she chose marching in place, dancing around her kitchen, and stretching to build strength and stamina.

A vegetarian eating pattern like hers presents unique challenges, such as getting enough iron, vitamin B12, zinc, and protein from plant sources. A thorough recall of her meals and snacks revealed a lot about the strengths and weaknesses of her eating style. Kathy's biggest mealtime struggle was extra servings of pasta, rice, or bread—"filler," as she called it—and favoring carbohydrates over protein. I used this information to focus our efforts. Reducing sodium, increasing portions of plant proteins, and increasing vegetables and fruits to take the place of fillers were among the food topics addressed at each of our visits.

Delving deeper into her meals revealed inadequate B12, iron, and zinc, requiring supplemental forms of these nutrients. Although I favor food first rather than reaching for a vitamin or mineral supplement, in Kathy's case, recent lab work from her doctor meant supplement recommendations were essential for health. Together we reviewed how to increase protein intake by incorporating tofu or beans into pasta. After five visits with Kathy, we adjusted calorie levels for weight control, and her energy improved. Supplementing iron and B12 made a notable difference in Kathy's daily stamina, and short bouts of waltzing around the kitchen island provided a jolt of energy and uplifted her spirit.

What I offer survivors is not magic; it is one part art, another part science. This implies that I must artfully pay heed to the stories that make up your life while allowing science to sift through files of evidence-based nutritional approaches. First, I must listen closely to what you tell me about your life. This is art, hearing the messages of survivorship struggle, pain, and triumph. Next, nutrition science is applied while acknowledging that you and others rarely have only a breast cancer diagnosis; you may also have heart disease, thyroid problems, diabetes, high blood pressure, or fibromyalgia. Overall, each of your health problems complicates the creation of an eating plan, which makes science a critical part of your nutrition. My greatest challenge and yours is the blending of the two. Arriving at that sweet spot where it all comes together is what it means to be in the pink.

Just for You: In the Pink Plate Plan

I chose to use the DGAs as the framework for my In the Pink Plate Plan because of their balance and the proven research behind them. Within the DGAs, I recognize opportunities to emphasize seven categories based on evidence from nutritional studies. This plan emphasizes food categories containing antioxidants, phytochemicals, vitamins, and minerals, which nutritional science has determined have the power to give you a healthier future. Too often, the seven categories highlighted are those that women, and in this case, breast cancer survivors, are deficient in daily.

- dark green vegetables
- red and orange vegetables
- beans, peas, and lentils
- fruits
- dairy foods
- seafood
- nuts, seeds, and soy products

Looking back at the notes gathered when I began this book, my priority was to present food categories in such a way that you, the survivor, will recognize that by paying heed to these foods, overall health improves, weight stabilizes, and you feel better. Throughout these chapters, you have learned how some foods have a greater health impact, and these are highlighted throughout the In the Pink Plate Plan with an asterisk (*) as an indicator that eating the recommended number of serving sizes has great nutritional benefits for you. A fine approach is to select one category at a time, working it into your daily and weekly eating plan with that lighter touch you need for the better health you seek.

Get Started Using the In the Pink Plate Plan

Years ago, food pyramids ruled the nutrition kingdom, and they still do; although the In the Pink Plate Plan is suited to display as a pyramid, it is not quite the same as those with which you are most familiar. Shown as an inverted pyramid, the In the Pink Plate Plan demonstrates the order of importance, with vegetables prominently at the top, then fruits, followed by grains, dairy, then protein foods and oils, making up 85 percent of the total calories per day until arriving at the tiny tip, the remaining 15 percent, assigned to calories for snacks and extras.

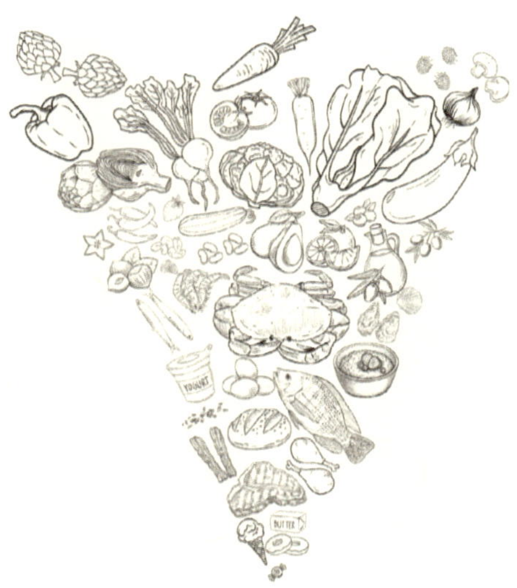

Review the plan first, noting food categories with daily or weekly guidance for serving sizes for each calorie level. The paragraphs below highlight examples of how to use the recommendations in daily or weekly ways for each category. The In the Pink Plate Plan is presented with nine calorie levels, ranging from 1,200 to 2,600. And, because a 1,500-calorie level suits the needs of many women, I will use a 1,500-calorie plan as an example throughout the rest of this chapter.

In the Pink Plate Plan

Calorie Level	1,200	1,400	1,500	1,600	1,800	2,000	2,200	2,400	2,600
Food group or subgroup	Daily Amount of Food from Each Group (Vegetable and Protein Groups have Subgroups)								
Total Cups of vegetables/day	1-1/2	1-1/2	1-1/2	2	2-1/2	2-1/2	3	3	3-1/2
Vegetable Subgroups in Weekly Amounts									
*Dark-Green Vegetables (cups /week)	1	1	1	1-1/2	1-1/2	1-1/2	2	2	2-1/2
*Red and Orange Vegetables (cups /week)	3	3	3	4	5-1/2	5-1/2	6	6	7
*Beans, Peas, Lentils (cups /week)	1/2	1/2	1/2	1	1-1/2	1-1/2	2	2	2-1/2
Starchy Vegetables (cups /week)	3-1/2	3-1/2	3-1/2	4	5	5	6	6	7
Other Vegetables (cups /week)	2-1/2	2-1/2	2-1/2	3-1/2	4	4	5	5	5-1/2
*Fruits (cups/day)	1	1-1/2	1-1/2	2	2	2-1/2	2-1/2	2-1/2	2-1/2
Total Grains (oz/day)	4	5	5.5	5.5	6	6	7	8	9
Whole Grains (oz /day)	3	3.5	4	4	4	4	5	6	7
Refined Grains (oz/day)	1	1.5	1.5	1.5	2	2	2	2	2
*Dairy (cups/day)	3	3	3	3	3	2	2	2-1/2	2-1/2
Protein Subgroups in Weekly Amounts									
Protein Foods (oz /day)	3	4	4-1/2	5-1/2	6	6-1/2	7	7-1/2	7-1/2
Meats, Poultry, Eggs (oz /week)	14	19	21	23	23	26	28	31	31
*Seafood (oz/week)	4	6	8	11	15	15	16	16	17
*Nuts, Seeds, Soy Products (oz /week)	2	3	3	4	4	5	5	5	5
Oils grams/day) (teaspoons/day)	(17)(4)	17 (4)	19 (5)	22 (5)	24(5)	27(5)	29(6)	31(6)	34 (7)
Calories for Snacks/Extras 15% of total calories daily	180	210	225	240	270	300	330	360	390

*Adapted from Dietary Guidelines for Americans 2020–2025. *Food groups important for survivors.*

Detoxifying Specialists: Vegetables and Fruits

Due to an abundance of detoxifying components, vegetables and fruits deserve a prominent place in this plan and, as such, appear at the top. Figuring out how to attain the recommended servings of fruits and vegetables may be confusing, especially with a mix of both daily and weekly recommendations.

To illustrate vegetable and fruit servings for 1,500 calories per day:

- **Red and orange vegetables, 3 cups weekly:** ½ cup of a red or orange vegetable 6 days per week, or one cup 3 days per week.
- **Fruits, 1.5 cups daily:** 1 whole orange, a generous handful of blueberries, and a low-sugar fruit cup.
- **Starchy vegetables, such as corn, potatoes, or lima beans**, **3.5 cups weekly:** ½ cup of a starchy vegetable daily or 1 cup 3 days of the week.
- After a review of the plan, you recognize that to meet these recommendations, vegetables and fruits are served at each meal. In fact, ideally, fruits and vegetables make up one-half of each meal, with grains and protein foods comprising the remaining half. Progress, not perfection, is the goal. Greater attention to the recommended servings for each of the vegetable categories and fruit increases the likelihood that your eating plan nudges you closer to better health.

Categories of Vegetables and Fruits

Dark Green Vegetables	Bok choy, broccoli, chard, collard greens, Romaine lettuce, spinach, watercress, taro leaves
Red-Orange Vegetables	calabaza, carrots, red/orange bell peppers, sweet potatoes, tomatoes, winter squash
Beans · Peas · Lentils	chickpeas, lentils, pinto, edamame, split peas, butter beans
Starchy Vegetables	breadfruit, cassava, corn, jicama, lima beans, plantain, white potato, taro root, yam, water chestnuts, yucca. Not Included: French Fries
Other Vegetables	asparagus, avocado, bamboo shoots, bitter melon, Brussels sprouts, cabbage, cauliflower, celery, cactus pads, cucumber, eggplant, kohlrabi, mushrooms, okra, onions, seaweed, snow peas, summer squash, turnips, tomatillos. Not Included: Onion Rings
Fruits	apples, Asian pears, bananas, berries (e.g., blackberries, blueberries, currants, huckleberries, kiwifruit, mulberries, raspberries, and strawberries); citrus fruit (e.g., calamondin, grapefruit, lemons, limes, oranges, and pomelos); cherries, dates, figs, grapes, guava, jackfruit, lychee, mangoes, melons (e.g., cantaloupe, casaba, honeydew, and watermelon); nectarines, papaya, peaches, pears, persimmons, pineapple, plums, pomegranates, raisins, rhubarb, sapote, and soursop.

Next Up: the Goodness of Grains

Although not as popular as vegetables and fruits for powerful phytonu-trients, grains, especially in unrefined forms, contain plenty of powerful disease-fighting components. Recall what you learned in "Puzzle Pieces" about the balance between whole and refined grains. For a 1,500-calorie plan, 5.5 ounces of grains are recommended. What might the combination of whole and refined grains look like in a daily plan?

- 1.5 slices of whole wheat bread (whole)
- one small muffin made with refined flour (refined)
- ½ cup cooked brown rice (whole)
- ½ cup whole wheat pasta (whole)
- five small woven wheat crackers (whole)

Notably, on this day, there are 3.5 whole and two refined servings of grains, therefore meeting the recommendation for balance. Aiming to balance whole and refined grains on most days of the week is suggested, with the understanding that some days this is not possible, like while traveling or visiting a relative.

Doing Dairy Daily

As you learned in "Puzzle Pieces," most Americans do not get enough calcium from dairy foods for a variety of reasons, and breast cancer survivors are no exception, despite the concerns for bone health and a concerted focus on calcium. Chapter 6 reviewed the 1,200 milligrams of calcium women need to maintain bone health, a priority for survivors, particularly those taking aromatase inhibitors. Here's an example of a commitment to getting three servings of dairy daily:

- a cup of milk at breakfast, a carton of low-sugar yogurt at lunch, and a generous handful of cheese on a salad or stew for dinner

Other foods, such as broccoli, salmon, white beans, tofu, and almonds, also contain calcium, although in lesser amounts than dairy. In the case of dairy, however, take note that on the plan, the recommended servings *decrease* to less than three servings as calorie needs increase beyond 1,800 calories because additional calcium is derived from a greater variety and quantity of foods.

Perfecting Protein

Like balancing the varieties of vegetables, fruits, and grains, perfecting protein implies mixing and matching both plant and animal protein foods. As presented in chapter 6, the iron, zinc, and B vitamins in beef, chicken, and pork support normal cell metabolism, and choosing from lower-fat cuts reduces saturated fats. And, following the discussions found in chapter 6 about the benefits of anti-inflammatory essential omega-3 fatty acids, it will not surprise you to see a recommended serving of seafood weekly.

Further, nuts and seeds, sometimes overlooked as sources of protein, also carry healthy fats, phytonutrients, and important vitamins and minerals, while soy has protective properties for heart health, diabetes, and cancer prevention. In fact, three ounces, or roughly a half cup, per *week* of nuts, seeds, and soy also deliver monounsaturated and polyunsaturated oils. A typical 1,500-calorie plan of twenty-one ounces of protein weekly could include:

- a small hamburger for dinner on Monday, chicken breast on Wednesday, and a small pork chop on Friday
- two eggs for breakfast on Monday and Friday
- a handful of nuts for a snack on Sunday, Tuesday, and Saturday
- salmon or tuna for lunch on Thursday and Sunday
- three-bean salad for lunch on Monday and Wednesday

Equally important, recall that mixing and matching protein foods means incorporating meatless meals made of beans, peas, or lentils one to two times per week to put the finishing touches on perfecting protein.

Choose Oils Like a Cavewoman

Popular topics among podcasters, food gurus, dietitians, and others are reducing or eliminating "seed oils," also known as omega-6 fatty acids, such as safflower, sunflower, canola, soybean, and corn oils. Rummaging for oils like a cavewoman, as described in chapter 6, sets the eating plan on point with these trendy discussions. You'll increase your omega-9 fatty acids with olive and avocado oils as well as omega-3 fatty acids from salmon and tuna. Using a handful of nuts for a snack will perfectly position you alongside the trend for reducing seed oils, too.

Wisely notice that nineteen grams of oil equals five teaspoons per day, and this includes the amounts contained in crackers, pan sprays, and home-baked goods, as well as the servings of nuts and seeds you eat. These add up quickly. Oils and fats have more calories per gram than carbohydrates or protein, so even the smallest amounts are high in calories. To set up your day like a skilled cavewoman needing five teaspoons of oils daily:

- half cup pasta tossed with one teaspoon of olive oil, a small low-fat muffin made with avocado or walnut oil (approximately one teaspoon per muffin), an egg fried in one teaspoon of olive oil, and a serving of salmon

Hidden oils are found in packaged foods, and most of these are omega-6 fatty acids, or seed oils, and should be eaten sparingly. Furthermore, the saturated fats found in butter, bacon, cheeses, ice cream, and candy are included in the daily tally.

A Look at a Day with the 85-15 Way

Think back to chapter 6 and recall how, when combined, the food groups discussed in the previous paragraphs make up 85 percent of all the calories you eat each day. The row at the bottom of each calorie level displays 15 percent of the total calories left over at day's end for snacks and extras. For a 1,500-calorie plan, that 15 percent equals 225 calories, which often is applied to a dessert or snack like:

- small ice cream bar
- two cookies
- slim sliver of pie or cake
- five crackers and a slice of cheese

Using the 15 percent of calories remaining at day's end to address uncomfortable evening hunger is a clever way to both reward and take care of yourself. And applying the Two Bite Rule to desserts and snacks allows you to indulge, even if less than you would like.

Selecting the Right Plan for You

This In the Pink Plate Plan is a breast cancer survivor's anti-inflammatory, cancer-fighting, plant-based eating pattern and was created as an invitation for you to practice the following ideas summarized throughout this book:

1. **Improve the quality of your eating pattern by choosing lean proteins, higher fiber from whole grains, and fruits and vegetables.**
2. **Focus on foods that are high in nutrient-density to support the health of your cells. Limit energy-dense, high-calorie foods that deliver few nutrients.**
3. **The combination of 1 and 2 will result in a modest 5–10 percent weight loss and improved nutritional health, thus lowering your risk of disease.**

Recall how calorie calculations serve as a starting point, or an estimation, for determining how much energy your body needs. A range of daily calories, for example, 1,600 to 1,700, acknowledges how you do not eat the same number of calories, nor does your body require the same energy from day to day. The number of servings increases as calorie needs increase, except in the case of servings of dairy foods, as noted above, which decrease as calorie needs increase.

For instance, a 1,500-calorie level requires three cups *weekly* of red and orange vegetables, but a 2,000-calorie level jumps to 5.5 cups. Additionally, observe how the calories for snacks and extras, the 15 percent, which is 225 for 1,500 calories, increase to 300 for a 2,000-calorie level. And as a gentle reminder: counting calories is not the goal; paying attention to getting closer to the recommended servings of each food group is the goal.

Estimate Your Calorie Needs

Calculating your calorie needs is not rocket science, nor is it a hard and fast answer to capturing the exact number of calories you need. It is an estimate. Using the following tool, estimate your calorie range to suit your desired approach for weight stability, loss, or gain.

Example:
Weight in pounds 175 ÷ 2.2 = 79.5 kilograms.
Now round it up to 80 kilograms.

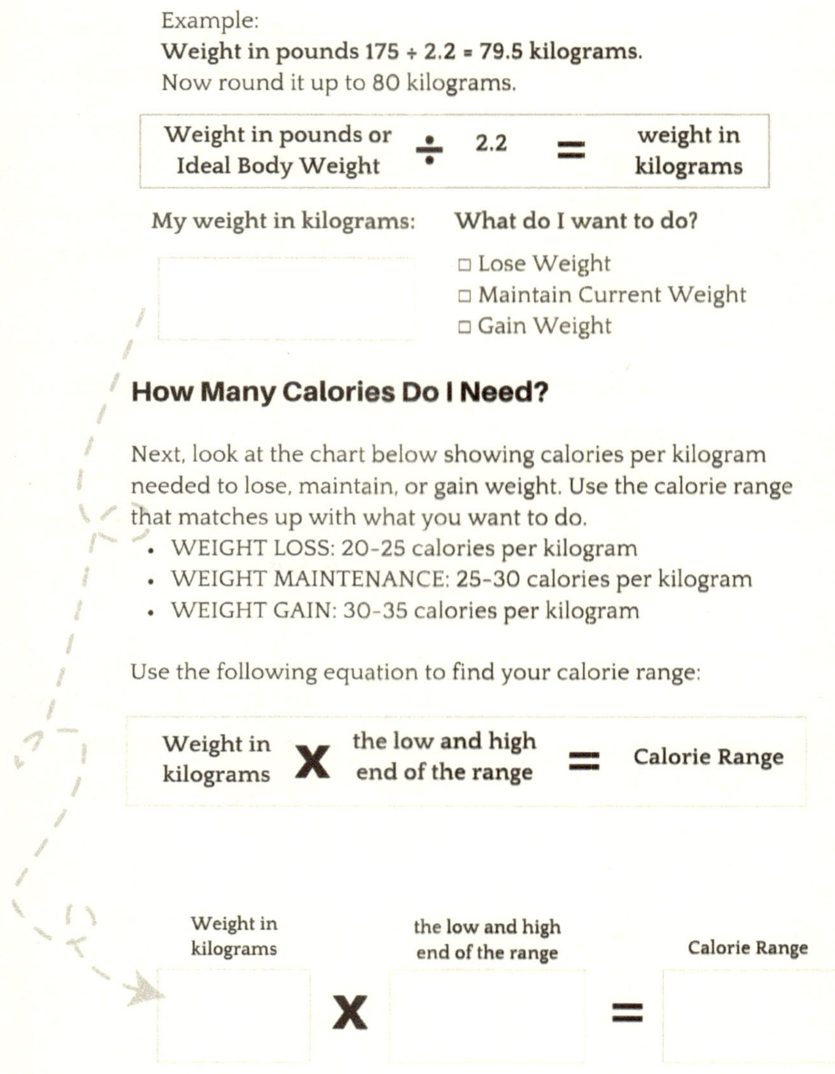

How Many Calories Do I Need?

Next, look at the chart below showing calories per kilogram needed to lose, maintain, or gain weight. Use the calorie range that matches up with what you want to do.
- WEIGHT LOSS: 20-25 calories per kilogram
- WEIGHT MAINTENANCE: 25-30 calories per kilogram
- WEIGHT GAIN: 30-35 calories per kilogram

Use the following equation to find your calorie range:

Enter both the low and high ends of the calorie estimates into the Build Your Own In the Pink Plate Plan. As an example, say that your calorie needs estimate shows a range from 1,450–1,645. Find the 1,500 and 1,600 columns to reflect this range of calories, then write, for example, 1.5–2 cups of fruits daily to show that, on average, you need 1.5 to 2 cups of fruits per day or ½ to 1 cup of beans, peas, or lentils each week. The calorie *range* allows for more realistic and workable flexibility within the food groups than sticking to an exact number. Write in the number of servings for each food group in the selected column:

	1500 Calorie Example	Your Calorie Level	Specific and Realistic Goals
Target for Food group or subgroup			
Total Cups of vegetables/day	1-1/2		
Vegetable Subgroups in Weekly Amounts			
*Dark-Green Vegetables (cups /week)	1		
*Red and Orange Vegetables (cups /week)	3		
*Beans, Peas, Lentils (cups /week)	1/2		
Starchy Vegetables (cups /week)	3-1/2		
Other Vegetables (cups /week)	2-1/2		
Fruits (cups/day)	1-1/2		
Total Grains (ozs/day)	5.5		
Whole Grains (oz /day)	4		
Refined Grains (oz/day)	1.5		
Dairy (cups/day)	3		
Protein Subgroups in Weekly Amounts			
Protein Foods (oz /day)	4-1/2		
Meats, Poultry, Eggs (oz /week)	21		
*Seafood (oz/week)	8		
*Nuts, Seeds, Soy Products (oz /week)	3		
Oils (grams/day)(teaspoons/day)	19 (5)		
Calories for Snacks/ Extras 15% of total calories daily	225		

*Adapted from Dietary Guidelines for Americans 2020-2025. * Food groups important for a survivor.*

Remember the ready, willing, and able exercise from chapter 2? Maybe after entering the recommended servings of each group, you discover that you are not ready, willing, or able to embrace the *entire* plan, but you believe you are ready to make a manageable change. Few, if any, of the survivors I have helped could overhaul the whole of their eating routines. Most of them are ready and maybe even willing to tweak some of their food choices but are not yet able to change everything about their eating styles. Start by favoring an easy goal to get started. Working on one food group at a time, in the Specific and Realistic Goals column, begin to consider your approach for incorporating the plan into your daily routines. Pause for a moment. A goal for you could be:

- "For this week, I will add two pieces of fresh fruit daily, one with breakfast and one more with lunch."

Or another one, such as:

- "Over the next two weeks, I will add leafy greens to my evening meal in the form of a salad."

These goals are specific, as in "this week," and realistic, as in one piece of fruit with both breakfast and lunch or adding leafy greens to evening meals. Stick to each doable goal for a week or two, then select another one and repeat this process until you are satisfied with your progress. Allow time for each food group adjustment to become a habit. Recall the importance of progress, not perfection, and patience in doing so.

Gradual additions to the seven priority food groups become a feathery, gentle way for you to trade old habits for improved ones. The point is that you choose the changes you are ready to embrace, the ones you may willingly endure and capably implement. Lining up all three—ready, willing, and able—is ideal, but if you wait until all three are intact, you may never begin.

The Higher Cost of Eating Well

Heaped atop the cost of cancer treatment co-pays, prescriptions, specialist visits, imaging tests, and unpaid bills is the high cost of eating well. Cancer cost experts have a term for the high cost of cancer treatment: financial toxicity.[93] I have witnessed the result of financial toxicity in the form of *nutrition insecurity*, which means the food budget affords sustenance but does not stretch far enough to fill your cart with the healthiest of foods.

Wanda, whom I introduced in "Glisten," appears at the top of my mind when I consider the price tag associated with eating well. Caring for her grandchildren and often providing meals for her adult children gobbled up all of Wanda's meager budget, with little left for her individual needs. "Four cups of vegetables a day?" she asked with a startled look on her face. Of course, my response was a resounding "Yes," with reminders about the cancer-fighting elements found in vegetables and the other food groups. Figuring out how to make this happen is another matter. Survivors, particularly those experiencing the financial toxicity of cancer, need to develop skills in cost-conscious shopping, preparing nutrient-dense foods on a tight budget, and limiting food waste. And, as Wanda could attest to, it is no easy feat.

Beef Substitutions for Meatless Meals

Meat Dish	Meatless Dish
Beef burrito with lettuce, tomato, and shredded cheese	Black bean burrito with lettuce, tomato, and 1 tablespoon shredded cheese
Meat-lover's pizza with pepperoni, sausage, peppers, and onions	Vegetable pizza with peppers, onions, and mushrooms
Loaded chili with beef, onions, beans, and tomatoes and topped with cheese and sour cream	Three-variety bean chili with tomatoes and onions, topped with reduced-fat cheese and sour cream

Following DGA recommendations can be pricey. A moderate weekly food bill for a woman fifty-one to seventy years old is $72.30.[94] To stay within food budgets, some survivors may choose less-nutritious foods, selecting processed foods and compromising nutritional well-being. In "Food as Medicine," you learned about the differences between nutrient- and energy-dense foods. Energy-dense foods, or unhealthy foods, tend to be cheaper and taste good. Processed foods like chips, frozen dinners and pizza, and packaged rice and noodle mixes are inexpensive and require less preparation than meals made with supplies from your pantry, but they are often high in salt and lower in nutritional quality. Meat is the highest-cost food group at the checkout, with fruits and vegetables a close second.

Mixing and matching meats and meatless meals weekly reduces not only saturated fats and introduces more nutritional variety, but it also costs less. Using canned tuna and salmon instead of fresh or frozen varieties offers similar omega-3 fatty acid content. Fresh, organic, frozen, and canned green beans have a wide spread of price points, but their nutritional value is the same.

Cost Comparison of Fresh, Frozen, and Canned Salmon And Green Beans

	Salmon	**Green Beans**
Fresh	$17.99 per pound	$1.79
Frozen	$7.49 per pound	$1.45
Canned	$4.39 for 14.75 ounces	$0.89 per 14.5 ounces

Cost based on supermarket prices as of August 2023

Fresh fruits and vegetables are costly, particularly if you select organic. Waste further increases the cost of fresh produce. A little-practiced approach is to adopt a motto of "fresh is sublime, frozen is divine, and canned is fine." Regardless of the form, the nutritional content is similar. Frozen produce retains all the nutrients and lasts much longer than fresh. Canned produce, like green beans and corn, has a long shelf life and provides a quick addition to meals. The companion journal for this book offers recipes using lower-cost food ingredients.

Here are my tips for improving the nutritional quality while stretching your food budget:

- **Plan your meals for the week.** Create a shopping list based on your healthy meal plan using low-cost, nutrient-dense recipes. Creating a list based on recipes and a quick look at pantry stock prevents last-minute unhealthy additions to your shopping cart. Grocery mobile apps offer valuable savings.
- **Cut up your own fruits and vegetables.** Although pre-cut produce can be more convenient, it can also be a lot more expensive.

- **Buy in bulk.** When possible, purchase food staples for the pantry and freezer in larger quantities. Consider buying your meat in bulk and freezing portions until ready to use.
- **Become a food label detective.** Ingredient lists and nutrition facts reveal the true story about foods, while labels are food marketing enticing you to buy foods by using words like *healthy*, *organic*, and *natural* to influence your purchase. Start by looking at the first three ingredients listed on the label for whole foods, and limit foods that have refined grains, added sugars, and hydrogenated/processed oils. Check the Nutrition Facts label for fats, added sugars, and nutrients.
- **Skip organic.** Choosing organic foods increases costs and does not guarantee nutritional advantages. However, if your food budget allows, organic foods are a good option as they do not contain genetically modified organisms (GMO), herbicides, pesticides, hormones, or glyphosates which have distinct non-nutritional advantages. Conventionally grown fruits and vegetables have the same nutritional value as organic foods, and keep in mind that when products are labeled as "contains organic ingredients," it does not mean they are nutritionally superior.
- **Make two, freeze one.** Embrace the practice of cooking once, eating twice. Save money by making two meal-size portions of healthy meals and freezing one for later. Embrace leftovers for both cost savings and better flavor for the next meal.

Because Wanda's work and family balance entailed the use of processed foods at meals, she designated lunch at work as her opportunity to get more whole grains and vegetables. Packing her brown bag with carrot sticks or other cut-up vegetables and fruits, a sandwich made with whole grain bread, and a carton of milk gave her satisfaction that one meal daily met her desire to eat better. Recognizing her limited ability to make sweeping changes to family mealtimes, Wanda made the best of her situation and employed what she was willing and able to do to eat as well as possible.

Finally, more than ever, Americans are eating meals in restaurants. In 2022, many households spent over $3,600 yearly dining out.[95] Not only is this a costly way to eat, but restaurant food choices tend to be higher in calories, saturated fats, and salt. A quick glance at the restaurant menu before you go saves money and calories and sets you up to select nutrient-dense choices before you are seated at the table. For information on how to find calories on restaurant menus, see the Resources list for this chapter.

More than Nutrition: Food Is Memories, Nostalgia, and Comfort

No two people use the same approach to changing eating habits. Family situations, ethnic cultures, household budgets, and traditions affect food decision-making. I learned this the hard way. Years ago, I met with Nadia, an Asian-Indian woman who asked for a meal plan after her treatment. I hurriedly gave her a tear-off sheet, made a few modifications, and shared it with her, and then she left. When she returned for another visit, she told me that the foods I had entered in the meal plan were not foods available in her pantry, nor did she regularly prepare any of those foods. That day, I learned from Nadia how each person is different and needs plans tailored to a unique culture. More sensitive ears and eyes would have helped me to help Nadia become more successful. Regardless of ethnicity or culture, you are more comfortable receiving nutritional guidance when food examples align with your preferences. A study exploring what drives African American women to adopt and stick to a plant-based eating plan showed that when recipes match cultural food choices, participants can sustain these lifestyle changes.[96] Flavors, spices, and ingredients are part of who you are, and embracing this fact helps you to avoid stumbling.

There is more to good nutrition than just the food in front of you, and there is more to your food than erasing the hunger in your belly. Foods do more than address a physical need for energy and nutrients; foods connect us to cultural identity, memories, nostalgia, and comfort. A strong connection to the familiar tastes, aromas, and textures of foods can reinforce your success in making changes. I grew up loving Mexican food (a cuisine not well-known for health-conscious eating). The flavors of green chile tortillas, cheese, beans, cilantro, and spicy meat taste like home to me. I simply cannot live without them, so using less cheese, whole wheat tortillas instead of white flour, brown rice, and more beans than meat allows me to sensibly eat Mexican foods.

Granting yourself permission to satisfy your taste buds with familiar flavors, textures, colors, and traditions is just as important as eating less sugars, fats, and overall calories. Culturally tailored recipes rooted in tradition are yet another way to pull us toward positive health habits. When you anchor an eating style with your ethnic and social food customs, the path to healthier eating occurs naturally and you are more likely to stick with it.

Like Nadia, you want familiar flavors and food preparation that aligns with your memories and culture. The In the Pink Plate Plan allows flexibility to tweak food groups with your preferences for fruits, vegetables, beans, spices, meats, and fish. Examples of my favorite flavorful, healthier cultural foods are:

- **Matoke** is a simple, healthy, and delicious one-pot East African dish made from stew meat and matoke (green banana). Served with kachumbari, a cucumber and tomato salad, this meal is easy to prepare and satisfying.
- **Shrimp pad Thai** served with rice vinegar, sliced cucumbers, and cilantro vinaigrette has less fat and fewer calories than more traditional versions.
- **Mexican fish tacos** with avocado-lime crema combines grilled tilapia, coleslaw, rice vinegar, and corn tortillas to lower the calories of other cheese-topped entrees.

- **Moroccan lentil stew with butternut squash**, a recipe in the accompanying journal, is a blend of warm Middle Eastern spices, creamy broth, and butternut squash sweetness. Comfort food, no matter your culture!

Great flavor, mouthfeel, and combinations of textures allow the stomach to tell the brain that you just ate something delicious and very satisfying. Healthy versions of familiar foods give you power over food.

Your Shade of Pink

Following the gray days of my diagnosis, I felt woefully ill-equipped to find my way back to health despite years of doing the same for thousands of others. Numerous heavy-handed attempts to escape the gray, foggy haze surrounding me were tossed aside after several days. Although I knew what I must do, I chose to remain in the same state of mind, stuck. Over the course of months that turned into a few years, I discovered the route of escape. Acknowledging the gratitude I felt for my treatment team, husband, and friends, the sadness lifted. Lapsed health habits were part of my past, and it was time to embrace better ones that would ensure a healthier future. I was ready to cast off my gray cloak. The time had come for me to work toward being in the pink.

For you, pursuing better health involves stepping into unfamiliar areas—honest evaluations of habits, new food choices and patterns, nutrition know-how, and the benefits of physical movement—and deciding which one to explore further and apply to your life. A desire to be healthier begs for *pink*, which is a combination of calm, tranquil white and passionate, fiery red. Quiet, persistent, and passionate, pink offers you kindness toward yourself and gratitude for the help of others. Playful and creative, pink lends you a durable devotion to get better and be better. With tender passion, pink reminds you of your desire to be at the pinnacle of your health.

Prior to my cancer diagnosis, I overlooked gentler methods for setting and achieving goals, yours and mine. More of a carpenter with a big hammer than an artist with a feathery brush, I employed a strong will and determination to address my ambitions. Today, as a member of the Breast Cancer Club, I see that cancer changes everything and methods that once worked are rendered useless. These days, I use a little finesse, applying a gentler touch to setting and achieving my health goals. What was once a favorite shade of mine, fiery coral, has been replaced by a preference for lighthearted bubblegum pink. This new favorite shade now reminds me to use a gentler approach, not a hammer. And not just toward myself but toward you, my fellow sister survivor.

Breast cancer survivors need more grace and less haste in their yearning for a healthier body and mind. Tenderly, remind yourself of the challenges you have overcome, the perseverance on display with each treatment completed, and the resiliency that emerged when you thought you could not go on. The tools throughout this book are designed for you to use a gentle stroke of brilliance when planning meals tailored to your needs or when seizing a moment of the day to move and swing your arms. Progress, not perfection, like an artist working on her canvas one detail at a time. Allow for smudges, spills, and little messes. A design planned with *your* vision of health and vitality is more likely to get you where you wish to be than one crafted around someone else's goals. Make it your own; be quiet or loud about the plan you have designed. Whether you prefer baby-soft pink or flashy fuchsia, wear your shade of pink with joy.

KEY POINTS

- The In the Pink Plate Plan spotlights seven food categories with evidence-based benefits for breast cancer survivors.

- Eating well is pricey; follow the tips for purchasing, storing, and preparing healthy foods while stretching food dollars.

- Embracing food as memories, nostalgia, and connection to family and culture allows you to appreciate it as more than sustenance.

ENDNOTES

1   "Cancer Treatment & Survivorship Facts & Figures 2022-2024," American Cancer Society, https://www.cancer.org/research/cancer-facts-statistics/survivor-facts-figures.html.

2   "The Survivorship Center Year 03 Executive Summary," American Cancer Society, https://www.cancer.org/content/dam/cancer-org/cancer-control/en/reports/summary-of-the-survivorship-center-year-three-activities.pdf.

3   Catherine Benedict et al., "Cost of Survivorship Care and Adherence to Screening-Aligning the Priorities of Health Care Systems and Survivors," *Transl Behav Med* 11, no. 1 (Feb 11, 2021): 132-142, 10.1093/tbm/ibz182.

4   "Survivorship Care Plans," American Society of Clinical Oncology, accessed April 14, 2023, cancer.net/survivorship/follow-care-after-treatment.

5   "Cancer Treatment & Survivorship Facts & Figures 2022-2024," American Cancer Society, https://www.fightcancer.org/policy-resources/costs-cancer-survivorship-2022.

6   Randy A Sansone and Lori A Sansone, "Gratitude and Well-Being: The Benefits of Appreciation," *Psychiatry* 7, no. 11 (November 2010): 18–22.

7   Robert A Emmons and Michael E McCullough, "Counted Blessings Versus Burdens: An Experimental Investigation of Gratitude and Subjective Well-Being in Daily Life," J Pers Soc Pyschol 84 (2003): 377–389.

8   Sally Helgesen and Marshall Goldsmith, How Women Rise: Break the 12 Habits Holding You Back from Your Next Raise, Promotion, or Job (Hachette Books, 2018), 17–22.

9   Stewart C Alexander et al., "Do the 5A's work when physicians counsel about weight loss?" Fam Med 43, no. 3 (2011): 179–84.

10   H Russell Searight, "Counseling patients in primary care," Am Fam Physician 98, no. 12 (2018): 719–728.

11   Emily B Falk et al., "Self-Affirmation Alters the Brain's Response to Health Messages and Subsequent Behavior Change," PNAS 112, no. 7 (2015): 1977–1982.

12   Matthew W Gallagher et al., "Resilience and Coping in Cancer Survivors: The Unique Effects of Optimism and Mastery," Cognit Ther Res. 43, no. 1 (February 2019): 32–44, doi:10.1007/s10608-018-9975-9.

13   Viktor E. Frankl, Man's Search for Meaning (Beacon Press, 2006), 104–105.

14   Kristi DePaul, "Managing Yourself: What Does It Really Take to Build a New Habit?" Harvard Business Review, February 2, 2021, www.hbr.org/2021/02/what-does-it-really-take-to-build-a-new-habit.

15   Brené Brown, Daring Greatly: How the courage to be vulnerable transforms the way we live, love, parent, and lead (Avery Publishing, 2015).

16   Frankl, 104–105.

17   Sarah J Hardcastle et al., "Motivating the Unmotivated: How Can Health Behaviors Be Changed in Those Unmotivated to Change?" Frontiers in Psychology 6 (2015): 835, doi.org/10.3389/fpsyg.2015.00835.

18   Phillipa Lally et al., "How Are Habits Formed: Modelling Habit Formation in The Real World," Europ J Soc Psych 40, no. 6 (2009): 998–1009.

19   Wendy Wood, Jeffrey M Quinn, and Deborah A Kashy, "Habits In Everyday Life: Thought, Emotion, Action," J Pers Soc Psychol 83, no. 6 (2002): 1281–97, PMID: 12500811.

20   DL Ronis, JF Yates, and JP Kirscht, "Attitudes, Decisions, And Habits As Determinants Of Repeated Behavior," Attitude, Structure and Function ed. Anthony R Pratkanis (Hilldale: Lawrence Erlbaum Associates, 1989): 213–239.

21 Ralph Ryback, "Why We Resist Change: How Behavioral Inertia Affects Success In Exercise And Weight Loss Goals," Psychology Today, January 25, 2017, www.psychologytoday.com/us/blog/the-truisms-wellness/201701/why-we-resist-change; Sally Helgesen and Marshall Goldsmith, "How Women Rise: Break The 12 Habits Holding You Back Form Your Next Raise, Promotion, Or Job" (Hachette, 2018), 29–44.

22 David Furman et al., "Chronic Inflammation in the Etiology of Disease Across the Life Span," Nat Med 25 (2019): 1822–1832, https://doi.org/10.1038/s41591-019-0675-0.

23 Mohammed S Ellulu et al., "Obesity and Inflammation: The Linking Mechanism and the Complications," Arch Med Sci. 13, no. 4 (2017 Jun): 851–863, doi: 10.5114/aoms.2016.58928; Laxmi S Mehta et al., "Cardiovascular Disease and Breast Cancer: Where These Entities Intersect: A Scientific Statement From the American Heart Association," Circulation 137, no. 8 (2018 Feb): e30–e66; Adenike O Eketunde, "Diabetes as a Risk Factor for Breast Cancer," Cureus 12, no. 5 (2020 May 7): e8010, doi: 10.7759/cureus.8010.

24 Carol J Fabian et al., "Favorable Modulation of Benign Breast Tissue and Serum Risk Biomarkers Is Associated With >10 percent Weight Loss in Postmenopausal Women," *Breast Cancer Res Treat* 142, no. 1 (2013): 119–132.

25 Ashish A Deshmukh et al., "The Association Between Dietary Quality and Overall and Cancer-Specific Mortality Among Cancer Survivors," NHANES III, JNCI Cancer Spectrum 2, no. 2 (April 2018): pky022, https://doi.org/10.1093/jncics/pky022.

26 Cheryl D Fryar, Margaret D Carroll, and Joseph Afful, "Prevalence of Overweight, Obesity, And Severe Obesity Among Adults Aged 20 And Over: United States, 1960–1962 Through 2017–2018," CDC (2020), https://www.cdc.gov/nchs/data/hestat/obesity-child-17-18/obesity-child.htm.

27 US Department of Agriculture and US Department of Health and Human Services, *Dietary Guidelines for Americans, 2020-2025*, 9th Edition, December 2020. Available at DietaryGuidelines.gov.

28 Reynalda Cordova et al., "Consumption of ultra-processed foods and risk of multimorbidity of cancer and cardiometabolic diseases: a multinational cohort study," *The Lancet* 35 (Nov 2023): doi: 10.1016/j.lanepe.2023.100771.

29 Colleen Gill, "Sugar and Cancer," Academy of Nutrition and Dietetics, Oncology Nutrition Practice Group, updated July 2014, https://www.oncologynutrition.org/erfc/healthy-nutrition-now/sugar-and-cancer.

30 Kevin C Maki, Mary R Dicklin, and Carol F Kirkpatrick, "Saturated Fats and Cardiovascular Health: Current Evidence And Controversies," *J Clin Lipidol* 15, no. 6 (2021): 765–772, doi: 10.1016/j.jacl.2021.09.049; American Heart Association, "Saturated Fat," www.heart.org/en/healthy-living/healthy-eating/eat-smart/fats/saturated-fats.

31 Anna Hopkins, "Study Probes Awareness of Alcohol's Link to Cancer," National Institute of Health, National Cancer Institute, (January 18, 2023): https://www.cancer.gov/news-events/cancer-currents-blog/2023/cancer-alcohol-link-public-awareness.

32 "Report Details Global Cancer Burden," National Institute of Health, National Cancer Institute, August 21, 2021, www.cancer.gov.

33 Marilyn L Kwan et al., "Alcohol Consumption and Breast Cancer Recurrence and Survival Among Women with Early-Stage Breast Cancer: The Life After Cancer Epidemiology Study," J Clin Oncol 28, no. 29 (2010): 4410–4416, doi: 10.1200/JCO.2010.29.2730.

34 "Alcohol: Drinking Increases Cancer Risk," American Institute for Cancer Research, March 31, 2021, www.aicr.org.

35 "Diet, nutrition, physical activity and cancer: a global perspective," World Cancer Research Fund/American Institute for Cancer, Continuous Update Project Expert Report, 2018.

36 Julie D Flom et al., "Alcohol Intake Over the Life Course and Mammographic Density," *Breast Cancer Res Treat* 117, no. 3 (2009): 643–51, doi: 10.1007/s10549-008-0302-0.

37 Hye-Yeon Koo et al., "Weight Change and Associated Factors in Long-Term Breast Cancer Survivors," *PLoS One* 11, no. 7 (2016): e0159098, doi: 10.1371/journal.pone.0159098.

38 "Cancer Stat Facts: Female Breast Cancer," Surveillance, Epidemiology, and End Results program (SEER), National Cancer Institute, www.seer.cancer.gov/statfacts/html/breast.html.

39 Anita M Arnold and Kerry Skurka, "Cardio-Oncology Care Delivered in the Non-academic Environment," Curr Treat Options Oncol. 23, No. 5 (2022 May): 762–773, doi: 10.1007/s11864-022-00978-w.

40 LL Lipscombe et al., "Incidence of Diabetes Among Postmenopausal Breast Cancer," Diabetologia 56 (2013): 476–483, doi 10.1007/s00125-012-2793-9.

41 Tengteng Wang et al., "Diabetes Risk Reduction Diet and Survival after Breast Cancer Diagnosis," Cancer Res 81, no. 5 (2021 Aug 1): 4155–4162, doi: 10.1158/0008-5472.CAN-21-0256.

42 L Kathleen Mahan and Sylvia Escott-Stump, "Eating to Detoxify," *Krause's Food and Nutrition and the Nutrition Care Process*, 13th ed. (Elsevier Inc., 2012), 438.

43 RJ Wurtman and JJ Wurtman, "Carbohydrate craving, obesity, and brain serotonin," *Appetite* 7 Suppl (1986): 99–103. doi: 10.1016/s0195-6663(86)80055-1.

44 Mya Nelson, "A Study Suggests Milk Increases the Risk of Breast Cancer, But AICR Experts Say Not So Fast," American Institute for Cancer Research, March 18, 2020, aicr.org.; Gary E Fraser et al., "Dairy, Soy, And Risk of Breast Cancer: Those Confounded Milks," *Intl Journ Epidemiol 49*, no. 5 (2020): 1526–1537, doi: 10.1093/ije/dyaa007.

45 Ni Shi et al., "Associations of Dairy Intake with Circulating Biomarkers of Inflammation, Insulin Response and Dyslipidemia Among Postmenopausal Women," J Acad Nutr Diet 121, no. 10 (2021): 1984–2002, doi: 10.1016/j.jand.2021.02.029.

46 Dietary Guidelines for Americans, 2020–2025.

47 "Recommendation on red and processed meat," American Institute for Cancer Research, updated January 29, 2020, https://www.aicr.org/resources/media-library/recommendation-on-red-and-processed-meat/.

48 Miguel A Lanaspa et al., "High Salt Intake Causes Leptin Resistance and Obesity in Mice by Stimulating Endogenous Fructose Production and Metabolism," *Proc Natl Acad Sci USA* 115, no. 12 (2018 Mar 20): 3138–3143; Richard Johnson, "Two surprising reasons behind the obesity epidemic: Too much salt, not enough water," *The Conversation*, August 22, 2022, https://theconversation.com/two-surprising-reasons-behind-the-obesity-epidemic-too-much-salt-not-enough-water-184128.

49   "Shaking the Salt Shaker Habit to Lower Blood Pressure," accessed August 8, 2023, www.heart.org/en/health-topics/high-blood-pressure; Andrea Grillo et al., "Sodium Intake and Hypertension," *Nutrients* 11, no. 9 (2019 Aug 21): 1970, doi: 10.3390/nu11091970.

50   "Salt in Your Diet: Use the Nutrition Facts Label and Reduce Your Intake," FDA, updated February 25, 2022, www.fda.gov/food/nutrition-education-resources-materials/sodium-your-diet.

51   Jay Rappaport, "Changes in Dietary Iodine Explains Increasing Incidence of Breast Cancer with Distant Involvement In Young Women," *Journal of Cancer* 8, no. 2 (2017): 174–177.

52   Carla Parry, Erin E. Kent, et al. "Cancer Survivors: A Booming Population," *Cancer Epidemiol Biomarkers Prev* 20 (2011): 1996–2005.

53   American Cancer Society, 2022, Preface.

54   "Cancer Statistics at a Glance," U.S. Cancer Statistics Working Group, based on 2022 submission data (1999–2020), Centers for Disease Control and Prevention, released November 2023, www.cdc.gov/cancer/dataviz.

55   American College of Sports Medicine, www.acsm.org; American Cancer Society, www.cancer.org; American Institute of Cancer Research, www.aicr.org.

56   Cheryl L Rock et al., "American Cancer Society nutrition and physical activity guideline for cancer survivors," CA Cancer J Clin. 72, no. 3 (2022): 230–262, doi.org/10.3322/caac.21719.

57   "Diet, Nutrition, Physical Activity, and Breast Cancer," World Cancer Research Fund/American Institute for Cancer Research, Continuous Update Project Report 2018, available at www.dietandcancerreport.org.

58   Carmen Fiuza-Luces et al., "Exercise Is the Real Polypill," *Physiology* 28 (2013): 330–358.

59   Barbara K Haas and Gary Kimmel, "Model for a community-based exercise program for cancer survivors: Taking patient care to the next level," *Journal of Onc Practice* 7, no. 4 (2022): 252–256.

60   Rowan T Chlebowski, "Nutrition and Physical Activity Influence on Cancer Incidence and Outcome," *Breast* 22, suppl 2 (2013): 530–7.

61   Martijn de Roon et al., "Effect of Exercise and/or Reduced Calorie Dietary Interventions on Breast Cancer-Related Endogenous Sex Hormones in Healthy Postmenopausal Women," *Breast Cancer Res* 20, no. 1 (2018 Aug 2): 81.

62   Robert James Thomas, Stacey A Kenfield, and Alfonzo Jimenez, "Exercise-Induced Biochemical Changes and Their Potential Influence on Cancer: A Scientific Review," *Br J Sports Med* 51 (2017): 640–644.

63   C Abbenhardt et al., "Effects of Individual and Combined Dietary Weight Loss and Exercise Interventions in Postmenopausal Women on Adiponectin and Leptin Levels," *J Intern Med* 274 (2013): 163–75.

64   Chat D Rethorst et al., "Considering Depression as a Secondary Outcome in the Optimization of Physical Activity Interventions for Breast Cancer Survivors in the PACES Trial: A Factorial Randomized Controlled Trial," *Int J Behav Nutr Phys Act* 20 (2023): 47, doi.org/10.1186/s12966-023-01437-x.

65   Elizabeth Anderson and Geetha Shivakumar, "Effects of Exercise and Physical Activity on Anxiety," *Frontiers in Psychiatry* 4 (April 23, 2013), doi.org/10.3389/fpsyt.2013.00027.

66   Robert James Thomas, 640–644.

67   Zhao Chen et al, "Fracture risk among breast cancer survivors: Results from the Women's Health Initiative Observational Study," *Arch Int Med* 165 (2005): 552–8.

68   Kerri M. Winters-Stone, PhD, et al., "Identifying Factors Associated with Falls in Postmenopausal Breast Cancer Survivors: A Multi-Disciplinary Approach," *Archives of Physical Medicine and Rehabilitation* 92, no. 4 (April 2011), doi:10.1016/j.apmr.2010.10.039.

69   Ewan Thomas et al., "Physical Activity Programs for Balance and Fall Prevention in Elderly: A Systematic Review," *Medicine* 98 (2019): 27(e16218).

70   Ezzeldin M Ibrahim and Abdelaziz Al-Homaidh, "Physical Activity and Survival After Breast Cancer Diagnosis," *Med Oncology* 28 (2011): 753–765.

71   National Cancer Institute, "For Women with Breast Cancer, Regular Exercise May Improve Survival," May 15, 2020, https://www.cancer.gov/news-events/cancer-currents-blog/2020/breast-cancer-survival-exercise.

72 Ana Paula Quixada et al., "Qigong Training Positively Impacts Both Posture and Mood in Breast Cancer Survivors with Persistent Post-Surgical Pain: Support for an Embodied Cognition Paradigm," *Frontiers in Psychology* 13 (2022), doi: 10.3389/fpsy.20232.800727.

73 Isobel Contento et al., "Developing a Diet and Physical Activity Intervention for Hispanic/Latina Breast Cancer Survivors," *Cancer Control* 29 (2022): 1–16.

74 Denise Spector et al., "A Pilot Study of a Home-Based Motivation Exercise Program for African American Breast Cancer Survivors: Clinical and Quality-Of-Life Outcomes," *Integrative Cancer Therapies* 13, no. 2 (2014): 121–132.

75 Kathryn Schmitz, "Moving Through Cancer: An Exercise and Strength Training Program for the Fight of Your Life," *Penn State Cancer Institute*, www.movingthroughcancer.com.

76 *Krause's Food and Nutrition and the Nutrition Care Process*, Chapter 5, 155.

77 AT Diplock et al., "Functional food science and defence against reactive oxygen species," *British Journal of Nutrition* 80, suppl 1 (1998): S77–S112; Marian Valko et al., "Free radicals and antioxidants in normal physiological functions and human disease," *International Journal of Biochemistry & Cell Biology* 39, no. 1 (2007): 44–84.

78 Amin Esfahani et al., "Health effects of mixed fruit and vegetable concentrates: a systematic review of the clinical interventions," J Am Coll Nutr 30, no. 5 (2011 Oct): 285–94, doi: 10.1080/07315724.2011.10719971; Ingrid Kiefer et al., "Supplementation with mixed fruit and vegetable juice concentrates increased serum antioxidants and folate in healthy adults," *J Am Coll Nutr* 23, no. 3 (2004 Jun): 205–11, doi: 10.1080/07315724.2004.10719362.

79 The Alpha-Tocopherol, Beta Carotene Cancer Prevention Study Group, "The effects of vitamin E and beta carotene on the incidence of lung cancer and other cancers in male smokers," *New England Journal of Medicine* 330 (1994): 1029–35.

80 Suong N.T. Ngo and Desmond B. Williams, "Protective Effect of Isothiocyanates from Cruciferous Vegetables on Breast Cancer: Epidemiological and Preclinical Perspectives," *Anti-Cancer Agents in Medicinal Chemistry* 21, no. 11 (2021): 1413–1430, doi: 10.2174/1871520620666200924104550.

81 Sin-Hye Park, Tung Hoang, and Jeongseon Kim, "Dietary factors and breast cancer prognosis among breast cancer survivors: A systematic review and meta-analysis of cohort studies," *Cancers* 13 (2021): 5329; A Heather Eliassen et al., "Circulating carotenoids and risk of breast cancer: pooled analysis of eight prospective studies," *J Natl Cancer Inst.* 104, no. 24 (2012 Dec 19): 1905–16; A Heather Eliassen et al., "Plasma carotenoids and risk of breast cancer over 20y of follow up," *Am J Clin Nutr* 101 (2015): 1197–1205.

82 Marcy J Balunas et al., "Natural products as aromatase inhibitors," *Anticancer Agents Med Chem* 8, no. 6 (2008 August): 646–682; Jean-Philippe Basly and Marie-Chantal Lavier, "Dietary phytoestrogens: potential selective estrogen enzyme modulators?" *Planta Med.* 71, no. 4 (April 2005): 287–94, doi: 10.1055/s-2005-864092.

83 D Aune et al., "Dietary fiber and breast cancer risk: a systematic review and meta-analysis of prospective studies," *Ann Oncol.* 23, no. 6 (2012): 1394–402, doi: 10.1093/annonc/mdr589.

84 Maryam S Farvid et al., "Fiber consumption and breast cancer incidence: A systematic review and meta-analysis of prospective studies," *Cancer* 126 (2020): 3061–3075, doi: 10.1002/cncr.32816.

85 Il-Sup Kim, "Current Perspectives on the Beneficial Effects of Soybean Isoflavones and Their Metabolites for Humans," *Antioxidants (Basel)* 10, no. 7 (June 30, 2021): 1064, doi: 10.3390/antiox10071064.

86 Yahui Fan et al., "Intake of Soy, Soy Isoflavones and Soy Protein and Risk of Cancer Incidence and Mortality," *Front Nutr.* 9 (March 4, 2022): 847421, doi: 10.3389/fnut.2022.847421.

87 Il-Sup Kim, "Current Perspectives on the Beneficial Effects of Soybean Isoflavones and Their Metabolites for Humans," *Antioxidants (Basel)* 10, no. 7 (June 30, 2021): 1064, doi: 10.3390/antiox10071064.

88 "Diet, Nutrition, Physical Activity, and Cancer: A Global Perspective Continuous Update Project Expert Report," *World Research Fund/American Institute for Cancer Research*, 41.

89 Marina S Touillaud et al., "Dietary lignan intake and postmenopausal breast cancer risk by estrogen and progesterone receptor status," *J Natl Cancer Inst.* 99, no. 6 (March 21, 2007): 475–86, doi: 10.1093/jnci/djk096; R Suzuki et al., "Dietary lignans and postmenopausal breast cancer risk by oestrogen receptor status: A prospective cohort study of Swedish women," *Br J Cancer* 98, No. 3 (Feb 2008): 636–40, doi: 10.1038/sj.bjc.6604175; Katharina Buck et al., "Meta-analyses of lignans and enterolignans in relation to breast cancer risk," *Am J Clin Nutr* 92, no. 1 (July 2010): 141–53, doi: 10.3945/ajcn.2009.28573.

90 "Saturated Fat," American Heart Association, www.heart.org/en/healthy-living/healthy-eating/eat-smart/fats/saturated-fats.

91 W Elaine Hardman, "(n-3) fatty acids and cancer therapy," *J Nutr* 134, suppl 12 (2004): 3420S–3430S, doi: 10.1093/jn/134.12.3427S; Carol J Fabian, Bruce F Kimler, and Stephen D Hursting, "Omega-3 fatty acids for breast cancer prevention and survivorship," *Breast Ca Research* 17, no. 1 (2015): 62, doi: 10.1186/s13058-015-0571-6.

92 Dawn L Hershman et al., "Randomized controlled trial of a clinic-based survivorship intervention following adjuvant therapy in breast cancer survivors," *Breast Cancer Research and Treatment* 138, no. 3 (April 2013): 795–806, doi: 10.1007/s10549-013-2486-1; Heather Greenlee et al., "Survivorship care plans and adherence to lifestyle recommendations among breast cancer survivors," *J Cancer Surviv* 10, no. 6 (Dec 2016): 956–963, doi: 10.1007/s11764-016-0541-8.

93 "Financial Toxicity (Financial Distress) and Cancer Treatment," National Cancer Institute, NIH, accessed August 23, 2023, https://www.cancer.gov/about-cancer/managing-care/track-care-costs/financial-toxicity-pdq.

94 "USDA Food Plans: Cost of Food, January 2024," USDA Food and Nutrition Service, accessed February 12, 2024, www.fns.usda.gov/cnpp/usda-food-plans-cost-food-monthly-reports.

95 "Average annual expenditures by major category of all consumer units and percent changes, Consumer Expenditure Surveys, 2019–22," Bureau of Labor Statistics, US Department of Labor, Consumer Expenditures in 2022, https://www.bls.gov/opub/reports/consumer-expenditures/2022/home.htm.

96   Nkechi Okpara et al., "'Food Doesn't Have Power Over Me Anymore!' Self-Efficacy as a Driver or Dietary Adherence Among African American Adults Participating in Plant-Based and Meat-Reduced Dietary Interventions: A Qualitative Study," *J Acad Nutr Diet* 122, no. 4 (2022): 811–824.

USEFUL RESOURCES

Introduction
The Survivorship Care Plan holds important information
about your treatment, the need for future check-ups and cancer
tests, the potential long-term late effects of the treatment
you received, and ideas for improving your health. www.
cancer.net/survivorship/follow-care-after-cancer-treatment/
asco-cancer-treatment-and-survivorship-care-plans

Chapter 1: An Attitude Of Gratitude
For more about defining gratitude, such as why it is important for
health and how to show gratitude daily, visit www.positivepsychology.
com/gratitude.appreciation.

A health coach can be a personal guide, partner, or cheerleader as you
implement lifestyle changes for greater health. Often offered through
corporate or insurance wellness programs, one may be recommended to

coach you through a chronic illness, like diabetes or heart disease. Most often, health coaches address issues that affect wellness, such as smoking, stress, nutrition, sleep, activity, and time management. To find a certified health coach, visit www.findahealthcoach.com.

Registered dietitians are uniquely trained to address nutritional needs with medical nutrition therapy and education. Most are highly trained in one or two areas of expertise. Some dietitians are certified in specialties like oncology, diabetes, and sports nutrition, and they work for hospitals, cancer clinics, fitness centers, and in private practices. To find a registered dietitian, visit www.eatright.org/find-a-nutrition-expert.

Chapter 2: Trade Old Habits For Better Ones

Author Nir Eyal reveals the hidden psychology driving you to distraction. Empowering and optimistic, this is the book that helps you design your time, create better habits, and live the life you want: *Indistractable: How to Control Your Attention and Choose Your Life*. Available at Amazon and other online retailers.

What women need to know about breast cancer and heart disease: https://www.heart.org/en/news/2020/02/19/what-women-need-to-know-about-breast-cancer-and-heart-disease

Breast cancer support groups, education, and fundraising: A go-to resource for clear, reliable, accurate, and up-to-date breast cancer information and community support. www.breastcancer.org

Helping women survive the trauma of cancer, one friend at a time: The mission of Breast Friends is to ensure that no woman goes through a diagnosis of cancer alone. We strive to be relevant, accessible, and inclusive of all people. Regardless of where you are on your journey, we are here for you. www.breastfriends.org

Pink Fund provides financial support to help meet basic needs, decrease stress levels, and allow breast cancer patients in active treatment to focus on healing while improving survivorship outcomes. A ninety-day grant program allows survivors to meet their critical expenses for housing, transportation, food, utilities, and insurance. www.pinkfund.org

The Susan G. Komen Foundation's mission is to save lives by meeting the most critical needs in communities and investing in breakthrough research to prevent and cure breast cancer. www.komen.org

Learn about cancer prevention, screening, treatment, and survivorship from the leading organization working to help people facing cancer. Find support, resources, services, and research from the American Cancer Society. www.cancer.org

For more information about the connections between breast cancer and diabetes: https://www.diabetes.org/diabetes-risk/prevention/diabetes-and-cancer

Groups on Facebook:
- Breast Cancer Awareness
- Breast Cancer Community: Support, Resources, and Discussion
- Hormone Positive Breast Cancer Support
- Kindred Spirits Warrior Women

Chapter 3: Food As Medicine

Emotional eating: Fellow breast cancer survivor and dietitian Cathy Leman offers help with emotional eating through The Peaceful Plate. www.cathyleman.com

Alcoholic beverages: More information on calories in alcoholic beverages. rethinkingdrinking.niaaa.nih.gov/tools/ calculators/calorie-calculator.aspx

Guidelines for drinking in moderation: Distilled Spirits Council of the United States. www.drinkinmoderation

Food and nutrition resources, including articles on anti-inflammatory foods: Harvard Health Publications. www.health.harvard,edu/staying-healthy/foods-that-fight-inflammation

Chapter 4: Puzzle Pieces

Calorie Counter by Fat Secret: Find great meal ideas, diet tools, community support, and more for free as you discover a world of healthy eating. www.fatsecret.com

Control My Weight app by Calorie King: www.calorieking.com

My Fitness Pal: MyFitnessPal is a smartphone app and website that tracks diet and exercise. The app uses gamification elements to motivate users. To track nutrients, users can either scan the barcodes of various food items or manually find them in the app's large preexisting database. www.myfitnesspal.com

Six Factors to Fit: Weight Loss That Works for You! Robert F. Kushner, MD; Nancy Kushner, MSN, RN; Dawn Jackson Blatner, RDN. Available at www.amazon.com.

To correctly measure your waist circumference:

- Stand and wrap a tape measure around your waist, just above your hipbones.
- Make sure the tape is horizontal around the waist.
- Keep the tape snug but not compressing the skin.
- Measure your waist just after you breathe out.

Or watch a YouTube video on how to measure your waist circumference. youtu.be/t4LYqIxWHQQ

Waist-to-hip ratio calculator: www.omnicalculator.com/health/waist-hip-ratio

Weight loss/gain/maintain calorie calculator, body mass index (BMI) tools, and more: www.calculator.net/calorie-calculator.html

Weight Watchers™: A global company headquartered in the US offering various products and services to assist in healthy habits, including weight loss and maintenance, fitness, and mindset such as the Weight Watchers comprehensive diet program. Online and mobile apps include tracking foods and exercise, Fit On exercise videos, recipes, and inspiration from other members. $20–$50/month. www.weightwatchers.com

Chapter 5: Glisten

12 yoga poses for bone health and strength: Basic, doable yoga poses for the beginner, based on Dr. Loren Fishman's Method for Avoiding Osteoporosis. www.youtube.com/watch?v=nrnn-ekrmas

Short, 5-minute activity bouts for all levels of fitness: Body Groove. www.bodygroove.com

Strength training for cancer patients and cancer survivors by Recovery Fitness: Improve your recovery and fitness with Exercise Specialist Carol Michaels as she leads you through safe movements and exercises to aid recovery and increase fitness levels. To order Carol's DVD, visit www.recoveryfitness.net and www.carolmichaels.com. DVDs also available on amazon.com.

Cancer Exercise Training Institute: An online guide to finding a certified cancer exercise trainer. https://www.thecancerspecialist.com/user-directory/

Cancer Fitness specialist: Find a trainer who specializes in helping persons with cancer by visiting the American College of Sports Medicine. https://www.acsm.org/get-stay-certified/find-a-pro

Casting for Recovery (CFR) provides healing outdoor retreats with fly fishing for women with breast cancer at no cost to the participants. https://castingforrecovery.org/

Effects of Exercise on Health-Related Outcomes in Those with Cancer: An infographic outlining evidence to support aerobic and resistance training exercise for cancer survivors. https://www.acsm.org/

Food & Fitness After 50: Eat Well, Move Well, Be Well by Christine Rosenbloom and Bob Murray, Academy of Nutrition and Dietetics. Eat Right Press, 2018.

Leslie Sansone leads east-to-follow walking videos for all levels: Leslie's One Mile Walking video can be found at www.youtube.com/watch?v=tW9IY48x1bc.

Livestrong® at the YMCA: In partnership with the Livestrong Foundation, the YMCA has developed a small-group twelve-week cancer survivorship program for those who are living with, through, or beyond cancer. Learn more about their specialized program and watch inspiring stories from survivors. https://www.ymca.org/what-we-do/healthy-living/fitness/livestrong

Moving Through Cancer Program: Worksheets to help you see how you can add more physical activity. https://www.exerciseismedicine.org/eim-in-action/moving-through-cancer/

More than just a workout, Nia exercise fills a void where traditional fitness programs fall short. A powerful fusion of dance, martial arts, and mindfulness practices, Nia is a holistic movement and wellness practice addressing each aspect of your life—body, mind, and soul. Nia has a class or program for everybody, regardless of age, health, or fitness level. Using a system of fifty-two simple moves, each Nia workout delivers full-body conditioning, leaving you energized, mentally clear, and emotionally balanced. www.nianow.com

Physical Activity and the Person with Cancer from the American Cancer Society provides general guidance about becoming more active at any level after a cancer diagnosis. Included are ways to be more active through daily chores and tasks and the importance of variety in your activity plans. www.cancer.org/cancer/survivorship/be-healthy-after-treatment/physical-activity-and-the-cancer-patient.html

Virtual fitness and Stand Up Str8: Exercise physiologist and certified personal trainer Ken Belveal offers workouts to alleviate back and neck pain through fitness. He has been helping clients for over thirty years to create a fit, healthy body before and after surgery. www.mobile-workout. com and www.standupstr8.com/

Step counters are an innovative and fun way to encourage more daily steps. There are many choices in step counters, such as: www.mypacer. com, www.myfitnesspal.com, Google Fit, Leap Fitness Step Counter, www.fitbit.com, pedometer by ITO Technologies, and apple.com.

To find a cancer rehabilitation and exercise program in your area, visit www.exerciseismedicine.org. Enter your search information in the Exercise Program Directory. Medical, community-based, and at-home programs are listed. Contact information is supplied so that you can reach out to a program coordinator to learn more.

CHAPTER 6: IN THE PINK

Breathe: You can use the Breathe app to help you relax and focus on your breathing. The app guides you through a series of deep breaths and reminds you to take time to breathe every day. Choose how long you want to breathe, then let the animation and gentle taps help you focus.

Healthy 10 Challenge: AICR's ten-week interactive program will help you build healthy habits to eat smarter and move more. http://healthy10challenge.org

How much calcium do I need? Use the Rule of 300 Tool from American Bone Health. https://americanbonehealth.org/nutrition/calcium-rule-of-300/

Karen Collins, registered dietitian and blog writer, takes nutrition information from daunting to doable. Many topics about cancer and other nutrition-related diseases appear on her site. www.karencollinsnutrition.com/

Free MyPlate tools include Shop Simple, Start Simple, Alexa My Plate, and more. https://www.myplate.gov/resources/tools

Noom is a behavior modification app that helps you build healthier habits to lose weight—the focus is on eating behaviors. Fees apply. www.noom.com

Real Plans: Meal planning, cooking, and shopping software. Mediterranean, vegetarian, and classic healthy eating patterns are included, and it costs about $40 monthly.

Mediterranean Diet Pyramids: The Mediterranean diet has been shown to help with heart disease, hypertension, cancer, and diabetes and is available for Asian, African, Hispanic, and vegetarian eating styles and more. An app is available for iPad and iPhone. There's a free version and a plan with a monthly fee to get access to all the features.

Oldways Preservation and Exchange Trust: Oldways is a nonprofit dedicated to improving public health by inspiring individuals and organizations to embrace the healthy, sustainable joys of the "old ways" of eating—heritage-based diets high in taste, nourishment, sustainability, and joy. The site includes food heritage pyramids for a variety of ethnic traditions, as well as videos and webinars. www.oldwayspt.org

Chapter 7: A Brighter Shade of Pink: In the Pink Plate Plan

Calories on the Menu: Information for consumers and nutrition facts for foods served in restaurants, with a free My Plate app. https://www.fda.gov/food/nutrition-education-resources-materials/calories-menu

Step to Health: A food pyramid devised by The Spanish Society of Community Nutrition includes the importance of socializing. www.steptohealth.com/get-know-new-food-pyramid

Healthy Eating Pyramid by the Harvard School of Public Health features physical activity at the base of the pyramid. www.hsph.harvard.edu/nutritionsource/healthy-eating-pyramid

Healing Foods Pyramid by University of Michigan author Monica Myklebust places fruits and vegetables at the base of this pyramid. www.canr.msu.edu › foodsystems › uploads › files › TheHealingFoodsPyramid.pdf

ACKNOWLEDGMENTS

BECAUSE OF THE THOUSANDS of breast cancer survivors whom I had the privilege of helping, *In the Pink* came to life in me. I can never thank enough those who taught me the hard lessons of listening more than speaking, but Robin was the first to get me to quiet my mind, close my mouth, and open my ears. An admission of gratitude to the appearance of three angels the day I was diagnosed: from that point forward, I had a new mission.

Thank you to:

Guy Hatch for tireless listening, reading, reflecting, and fishing.

Natasha Garnett for setting my tone. Maura Harrigan, MS, RD, for foundational direction. My ladies, you know who you are: SD, KG, LR. Kathy Peer for addressing the power of words. Cindy and Noah Wood for hearing me out. Jenny Fulton for stepping in. Janice Carr for walking as a fellow survivor and cancer professional. Jen, Lindy, and Cameron—for reminding me to go big or go home.

Although it is impossible to individually thank the teams of oncologists, surgeons, pathologists, radiation therapists, oncology nurses, social workers, dietitians, and office staff for an education taught through experience, I am indebted to these dedicated professionals who claim a passion for cancer care. I was privileged to belong to this group.

And to my publishing team:

Alexandra O'Connell, for expert organization, wordsmithing, and support for my project.

Graphics and Layout by Victoria Wolf of Wolf Design and Marketing and Betty Lok of Betty Wonderful, LLC

Kiki Ringer of KLR Literary, for steadying the course and walking me away from the precipice.

ABOUT THE AUTHOR

LAURIE HATCH, RD, is a certified cancer dietitian with nearly two decades of experience providing nutrition care for persons with cancer. She is a breast cancer survivor with a passion and drive to give other survivors the healthier life they want and deserve. She is a former fitness instructor, lifelong outdoor enthusiast, and devoted reader of all things related to breast cancer. Laurie, a mother of three and grandmother, lives with her husband 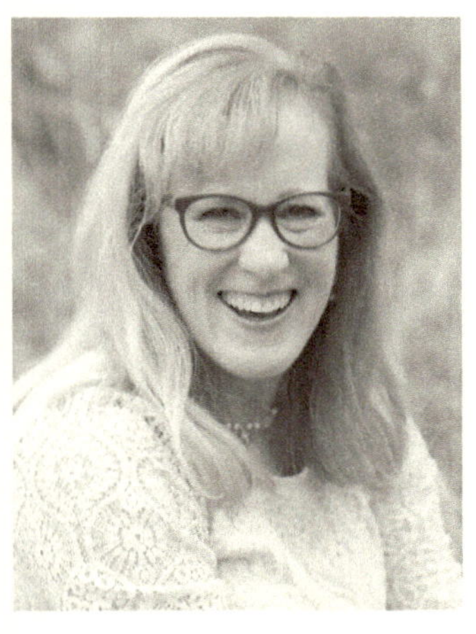 near Denver, Colorado. You can find Laurie online at foodismedicinerd.com, email via foodismedicinerd@gmail.com, on Facebook @lauriehatchfoodismedicinerd, and Instagram @foodismedicinerd_cancer.